PHYSICA DE HUMANO CORPUS

Physics of the Human Body

SENIOR EDITOR

RICHARD JUSTIN INGEBRETSEN MD PHD
DEPARTMENT OF PHYSICS AND ASTRONOMY
UNIVERSITY OF UTAH

EDITOR

JUSTIN S. COLES
DEPARTMENT OF PHYSICS AND ASTRONOMY
UNIVERSITY OF UTAH

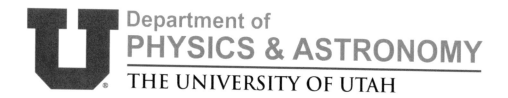

Department of
PHYSICS & ASTRONOMY
THE UNIVERSITY OF UTAH

COPY EDITOR

JULIE ROBERTS

COVER

DILLON JENSEN

RESEARCH

P. EGAN ANDERSON

WILLIAM GOCHNOUR

EDITION 1.2 COPYRIGHT (C) 2013

BY TRAVEL MEDICINE PRESS

ISBN: 0615776000

ISBN 13: 9780615776002

CONTRIBUTORS

P. Egan Anderson
University of Utah
Department of Physics and Astronomy
Salt Lake City, Utah

Desmond James Barker
University of Utah
Department of Physics and Astronomy
Salt Lake City, Utah

Adam Beehler
University of Utah
Lecture Demonstration Specialist
Department of Physics and Astronomy
Salt Lake City, Utah

Julie Bolick MS, RD, CD, CLS, FNLA
LiVe Well Center
Salt Lake City, Utah

Landon Coles
University of Utah
Department of Physics and Astronomy
Salt Lake City, Utah

Justin S. Coles
University of Utah
Department of Physics and Astronomy
Salt Lake City, Utah

Niaree Davis
University of Utah
Department of Physics and Astronomy
Salt Lake City, Utah

Gregory Ellis MD
The Center for Change
Medical Director, Psychiatry
Salt Lake City, Utah

James Ellis
University of Utah
Department of Physics and Astronomy
Salt Lake City, Utah

William Gochnour
University of Utah
Department of Physics and Astronomy
Salt Lake City, Utah

Peter Haight
Utah State University
Logan, Utah

Richard J. Ingebretsen MD, PhD
University of Utah
Department of Physics and Astronomy
University of Utah School of Medicine
Salt Lake City, Utah

Stein Ingebretsen
Medical Student
Rosalind Franklin University
Chicago, Illinois

Randy Jensen MD, PhD
University of Utah
Department of Neurosurgery
University of Utah School of Medicine
Salt Lake City, Utah

Daniel Oldroyd
Medical Student
Wake Forest University School of Medicine
Winston-Salem, North Carolina

Remington Plewe
University of Utah
Department of Physics and Astronomy
Salt Lake City, Utah

G. Andrew Wright
University of Utah
Department of Physics and Astronomy
Salt Lake City, Utah

TABLE OF CONTENTS

CHAPTER 1:

Energy

From sitting, to walking, to even thinking, all activities in the body require a significant amount of energy to function properly. In this chapter we will discuss the basic energy forms that are found in the body, how they are harnessed, and how this energy is used.

Carbohydrates

A carbohydrate is an organic compound that consists only of carbon, hydrogen, and oxygen. The term is a synonym of saccharide. The carbohydrates (saccharides) are divided into four chemical groupings: monosaccharides, disaccharides, oligosaccharides, and polysaccharides. In general, the monosaccharides and disaccharides are commonly referred to as sugars. The names of the monosaccharides and disaccharides very often end in the suffix –ose. For example, blood sugar is the monosaccharide glucose, table sugar is the disaccharide sucrose, and milk sugar is the disaccharide lactose. Carbohydrates perform numerous roles in living organisms. Polysaccharides serve for the storage of energy (starch and glycogen), and as structural components (cellulose in plants and chitin in arthropods). Ribose is an important component of coenzymes such as ATP and the backbone of the genetic molecule known as RNA. The related deoxyribose is a component of DNA. In food science, and in many informal contexts, the term carbohydrate often means any food that is particularly rich in the complex carbohydrate starch (such as cereals, bread, and pasta) or simple carbohydrates, such as sugar found in candy, jams, and desserts.

All living organisms need foodstuffs to continue living, or to continue their lives and keep surviving, thriving and growing. There are three types of foods: sugars, fats and proteins. All are vital and have nutritional value to humans as the donors of building materials and providers of energy.

Sugars

Sugars are our main energy source and are found in almost all food. Sugars can be divided into two groups: the simple sugars (monosaccharides) and complex sugars (disaccharides), which are composed of multiple units of monosaccharides.

Glucose, fructose and galactose are examples of monosaccharides, with the general formula $C_6H_{12}O_6$. These sugars occur naturally in fruits and plants as the primary product of photosynthesis. This is the process where organisms absorb energy from sunlight and use it to produce sugar and other organic compounds such as fats and proteins.

Most carbohydrates that we eat are converted into glucose during digestion. This is the form of sugar that is transported around the bodies of humans in the bloodstream.

Fats

Fats are energetically the most concentrated of all sustenance materials. They are found in both plants and animals and provide these living organisms with energy. Thanks to the chemical structure of fats, they can provide organisms with the greatest amount of energy possible from the least amount of matter. Because most animals, including humans, need to keep a store of energy for times when it is needed, these stores of fat cannot be shed easily. In other words, it is difficult to lose unwanted weight, or fat, because the body is programmed to hold onto it. Plant fats are naturally occurring liquids, while animal fats are solids at room temperature.

Proteins

Proteins are composed of long chains of amino acids. Amino acids are molecules composed of one type of organic compound called an amino group and another one called a carboxylic group. While it is not important to understand the details, it is interesting to note that proteins can be composed of more than 200 amino acids, most of which are water-soluble. Because proteins are very important to the function of the body, they are rarely used as an energy source.

Digestion

When we eat foods like bread, meat, and vegetables, they are not yet in a form that the body can use as nourishment. Our food and drink must be changed into smaller molecules of nutrients before they can be absorbed into the blood and carried to cells throughout the body. Digestion is the process by which food and drink are broken down into their smallest parts so that the body can use them to build and nourish cells and to provide energy.

Digestion involves the mixing of food, its movement through the digestive tract, and the chemical breakdown of the large molecules of food into smaller molecules. Digestion begins in the mouth, when we chew and swallow, and is completed in the small intestine. The chemical process varies somewhat for different kinds of food. It takes around 24 hours for food to move through our system.

The first major muscle movement occurs when food or liquid is swallowed. Although we are able to start swallowing by choice, once the swallow begins, it becomes involuntary and proceeds under the control of the nerves.

The food then enters the stomach, which has three mechanical tasks to do. First, the stomach must store the swallowed food and liquid. This requires the muscle of the upper part of the stomach to relax and accept large volumes of swallowed material. The second job is to mix up the food, liquid, and digestive juice produced by the stomach. The lower part of the stomach mixes these materials by its muscle action. The third task of the stomach is to empty its contents slowly into the small intestine.

After the stomach empties the food and its juice into the small intestine, the juices of two other digestive organs mix with the food to continue the process of digestion. One of these organs is the pancreas. It produces a juice that contains a wide array of enzymes to break down the carbohydrates, fat, and protein in our food.

The liver produces yet another digestive juice—bile. The bile is stored between meals in the gallbladder. At mealtime, it is squeezed out of the gallbladder into the bile ducts to reach the intestine and mix with the fat in our food. The bile acids dissolve the fat into the watery contents of the intestine, much like detergents that dissolve grease from a frying pan.

Energy in the Body

Food contains a lot of energy that is just waiting to be released. The body is very good at taking energy from the food we eat. The body absorbs nearly 95 percent of all energy stored in food. After eating a meal, the food that we eat is oxidized—meaning it loses electrons, which have a lot of energy. This process of oxidizing food, or obtaining electrons, is the way that we harness energy within the body to do work. The oxidation process takes place in the cells of the body and requires oxygen to accept or take the electrons from food. It is called the metabolic pathway, but sometimes it is referred to simply as metabolism. This process begins as soon as we consume some sort of food. Almost immediately, saliva within our mouths, along with fluids along the digestive tract, begins breaking down large food molecules into more manageable-sized molecules. These molecules will ultimately be broken down to release many types of substances within the body, but perhaps the most important substance that will come from this digestive process is glucose. The rate of energy production from the metabolic pathway is called the metabolic rate. Because the metabolic process requires oxygen, oxygen consumption increases while it is being performed.

Glucose—$C_6H_{12}O_6$—is the most common sugar and the principal source of energy for our body and brain. The oxidation reaction of glucose can be written as follows:

$$C_6H_{12}O_6 + 6O_2 \rightarrow 6H_2O + 6CO_2 + ATP$$

Another way to write it is like this:

$$Glucose + oxygen \rightarrow water + carbon\ dioxide + energy$$

So what is ATP? ATP stands for adenosine triphosphate. Cells require chemical energy for three general types of tasks: to drive metabolic reactions that would not occur automatically; to transport needed substances across membranes; and to do mechanical work, such as moving muscles. ATP is not a storage molecule for chemical energy—that is the job of carbohydrates, such as glycogen, and fats. When the cell needs energy, these storage molecules are converted into ATP, which then transports this chemical energy within cells.

The process to create ATP does not occur instantly, but rather through a process called sugar metabolism, which is made up of three parts:

1. Glycolysis
2. The Krebs cycle
3. The electron transport chain

The basics of each of these parts are not hard to understand. However it is important to note that what is discussed here is somewhat superficial, when in reality there are much more complex mechanisms at work.

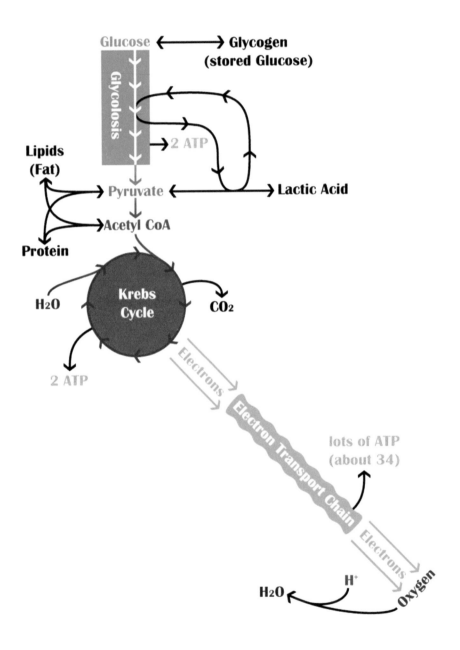

Glycolysis

The first step is called glycolysis, meaning "the splitting of sugar." Glycolysis is a metabolic pathway itself that is made up of 10 steps, all of which take place in the cytosol of cells in all living organisms. The process converts one molecule of glucose into two molecules of pyruvate, generating energy in the form of two net molecules of ATP. Four molecules of ATP are actually produced, but two are consumed in the process. It does not require oxygen, so it can function under anaerobic (no oxygen) conditions—and it happens quickly, within seconds. This is important, because it means that if you have to move quickly, for whatever reason, and you don't have oxygen but need ATP, you will get it quickly, but only in small amounts. This is also the reason why people will often look for a candy bar late in the day—so that they can get a shot of sugar rapidly, giving a quick blast of ATP. The end product of glycolysis is pyruvate.

The Krebs Cycle

The second step of sugar metabolism is called the Krebs cycle. It occurs in the mitochondria of every cell. It is named after Hans Adolf Krebs, the scientist who first identified it. The Krebs cycle does not occur very quickly compared to glycolysis and will not happen unless there is abundant oxygen present. Pyruvate does not enter the Krebs cycle directly. Instead, pyruvate advances forward into a coenzyme called Acetyl CoA, which then moves into the Krebs cycle. This is one reason why it is important to warm up when exercising so that you can get oxygen out to the cells, allowing this important step to advance.

Unlike glycolysis, which has a distinct starting and ending point, the Krebs cycle has no starting or ending point because it is cyclic (see diagram). This cycle churns around and around, two times for each molecule of Acetyl CoA, and gives two molecules of ATP each time around. The purpose of the Krebs cycle is to extract electrons from molecules that originally were in glucose. These electrons will ultimately enter the final phase of sugar metabolism and create ATP.

The Electron Transport Chain

The third step is called the electron transport chain and also occurs in the mitochondria of the cell in the electron transport chain. During this step, the electrons that were extracted from molecules in the Krebs cycle enter next into what is called the electron transport chain. The electron transport chain is located on the inner membrane of the mitochondria. The purpose of the electron transport chain is to harness the energy of each electron to make ATP. The movement of the electrons through the chain releases energy that creates ATP from ADP (adenosine diphosphate). This process needs lots of oxygen to accept the electrons after they have given up their energy. In fact, all of the oxygen that we breathe is utilized in this final step of the creation of ATP. The electron transport chain yields around 34 molecules of ATP, but the exact number of ATP produced depends upon the conditions in the cell.

Glycolysis occurs when there is no oxygen present. The Krebs cycle and the electron transport chain occur only when two conditions are present: there has to be abundant oxygen, and the body must be exercising or performing some sort of action. The byproducts of sugar metabolism are carbon dioxide and some water. This means, that as the equation above states, we eat food to get energy, we breathe in oxygen to accept electrons, and then we breathe out carbon dioxide, which is a waste product of the electron transport chain.

The Oxygen Debt

Oxygen is the ultimate electron acceptor. The blood needs oxygen continuously for ATP to be created in the electron transport chain. The amount of oxygen required is determined by how quickly the tissues are using it. If oxygen is available to the tissues, then ATP will always be created. If oxygen delivery is unable to keep up with demand, then the electrons get jammed up in the electron transport chain and the process stops. Fortunately, cells have a way to avoid this disaster. In a creative way, they convert pyruvate into a substance called lactic acid. There is an enzyme byproduct of this conversion, which moves step 6 (of the 10 steps) in glycolysis forward, rapidly creating two ATP molecules. This will give a person a rapid burst of energy when there is little oxygen present. An example would be a person running rapidly after a bus. Energy is provided by glycolysis through the production of ATP via the creation of lactic acid. After catching the bus, this person is completely out of breath and will be for some time; the heart rate will be high as well until the lactic acid produced is converted back into pyruvate. The next day, the runner's muscles will ache because lactic acid burns the tissue.

The ability to create ATP in this manner allows muscles and other tissues to continue working even when the availability of oxygen is low. However, this does not mean that we can live without oxygen. For one thing, only a tiny amount of ATP is created—only about five percent of the ATP that is normally used by the body. The production of lactic acid is not good for the cells. It leads to muscle cramps and burning. It also has a tendency to leak into the bloodstream, thereby interfering with proper cell function. So the body gets rid of lactic acid as soon as oxygen becomes available. As soon as the amount of oxygen returns to normal, lactic acid is converted back into pyruvate, which then moves forward normally into the Krebs cycle. This process of converting lactic acid back into pyruvate is called the oxygen debt. You will notice this when after a short run or burst of exercise you are out of breath for some time and your heart rate remains high as the body converts lactic acid back into pyruvate. When exercising, eventually people will become fatigued to the point that they cannot exercise any longer until the oxygen debt has been addressed by resting and breathing deeply. Deep breathing allows the body to re-oxygenate the blood, make more ATP, and break down lactic acid. After an adequate rest period, it will be possible to engage in physical activity again, although people may find that they will fatigue more quickly with a second round of exercise unless they have recovered completely. In review, if a person is exercising, has glucose, but has no oxygen, then the body forms lactic acid to create a limited amount of ATP for a brief period of time.

Formation of fat and proteins

What happens if the body has glucose, has enough oxygen but is not exercising? For example, what happens when you sit down, watch TV and eat a lot of carbohydrates such as potato chips? In this situation, the body will not create ATP since it is not needed. Instead, it will take pyruvate and Acetyl CoA and convert them first into fat and then into proteins. In this manner the body stores energy for future use. The opposite occurs when the supply of glucose is scarce. The body can break down fats and even proteins and return them to the metabolic pathway to be used as energy. The sum of this is very simple. If you eat carbohydrates without exercising, the body will create fat; if you exercise without eating carbohydrates, the body will utilize fats.

Basal Metabolic Rate (BMR)

So how much energy do we need? Even when we are at rest we consume energy. This rate of consumption, called the basal metabolic rate, or BMR for short, is the amount of energy needed to perform minimal body functions such as breathing or pumping of the heart under resting conditions. It is also sometimes referred to as the resting metabolic rate or RMR, but it is the same thing.

In order to keep a constant weight, an individual must consume just enough food to provide for basal metabolism plus physical activities. This means that eating too little results in weight loss, while a diet in excess food will cause an increase in body fat and therefore weight.

The metabolic rate depends primarily on three things. The first is the thyroid gland, which makes and stores hormones that help regulate the heart rate, blood pressure, body temperature, and the rate at which food is converted into energy. Thyroid hormones are essential for the function of every cell in the body. The thyroid gland is located in the lower part of the neck, below the Adam's apple, wrapped around the trachea. It has the shape of a butterfly.

The second factor that affects metabolic rate is the temperature of the body due to the fact that most chemical processes are temperature dependent. A small change in temperature can produce a profound change in the rate of chemical reactions. That is why when we participate in physical activities such as exercise or sporting activities, our bodies use more energy than when at rest. For example, if the body temperature changes by 1° centigrade, there is a change of about 10% in the basal metabolic rate. It is for this reason that hibernating at a low body temperature is advantageous to an animal or why some surgeries require lowering a patient's temperature to reduce oxygen consumption, as metabolism requires oxygen.

The third factor is body surface area. Much of our energy is given off as heat from our skin. Therefore large animals such as elephants have huge BMR's, while little animals such as a mouse have small BMR's.

Humans are not efficient users of energy. Usually about 90% of our energy is lost to heat. That is in contrast to home furnaces, which are about 95% efficient. Car engines are about 38% efficient. The rest of the energy is lost from the body as heat. The equation for efficiency of the human body as a machine is:

$$Eff = \frac{Work\ done}{Energy\ consumed}$$

There are some activities that are more efficient. Cycling, for example, can cause the body to reach an efficiency level of about 25%. The efficiency of the body also influences the maximum work capacity of the body. For short periods of time the body can perform at high power levels, but for long-term efforts the body is more limited for high-intensity levels.

What is a person's basal metabolic rate? There are a number of apps, web sites, and charts that will help you to determine this.

MEN				WOMEN		
Height (feet)	RMR Range	Mean		Height (feet)	RMR Range	Mean
5'4"	1200-1600	1400		5'1"	1120-1350	1240
5'5"	1275-1685	1480		5'2"	1135-1370	1255
5'6"	1340-1750	1550		5'3"	1155-1390	1275
5'7"	1410-1820	1610		5'4"	1195-1430	1315
5'8"	1480-1890	1680		5'5"	1235-1470	1355
5'9"	1550-1960	1750		5'6"	1270-1500	1390
5'10"	1615-2030	1815		5'7"	1310-1550	1430
5'11"	1685-2095	1885		5'8"	1350-1585	1470
6'0"	1750-2165	1950		5'9"	1370-1600	1490
6'1"	1820-2235	2020		5'10"	1410-1650	1530
6'2"	1890-2300	2100		5'11"	1450-1685	1570
6'3"	1960-2370	2160				
6'4"	2030-2440	2230				

Heat Loss from the Body

We just read that heat is 'lost' from the body. How does this occur? First off, it is important to know that there is no such thing as 'cold.' We commonly refer to something being cold, but what we really mean is that something just has less heat. Heat is transferred from one object to another. This means that if you hold ice up to your skin, you are not transferring cold into the body; you are transferring heat out of the body.

The body regulates temperature like a furnace. It is constantly producing heat and then dispersing it through various processes. Heat can be lost through three processes: conduction, convection, and radiation. Evaporation is also a method by which heat is lost, but it uses all three of the processes listed above. **Conduction** is the process of losing heat through physical contact with another object or body. For example, if you were to sit on a metal chair, the heat from your body would transfer to the cold metal chair. **Convection** is the process of losing heat through the movement of air or water molecules across the skin. The use of a fan to cool off the body is one example of convection. The amount of heat loss from convection is dependent upon the airflow or the water flow over the skin. Convection is where the wind-chill factor is truly relevant. **Radiation** is a form of heat loss through infrared rays. This involves the transfer of heat from one object to another, with no physical contact involved. For example, the sun transfers heat to the earth through radiation. Another process of heat loss is evaporation. **Evaporation** is the process of losing heat through the conversion of water to gas (evaporation of sweat). It utilizes convection, conduction and radiation. In order for evaporation to work, sweat on the skin must evaporate, not just drip off onto the floor.

Exercise

Exercise changes the body's metabolic needs. Oxygen demands soar and the output of the heart increases by increasing the heart rate. The systolic blood pressure will increase while the diastolic blood pressure does not rise too much. The body will increase sweating as it tries to lose excess heat through evaporation. There are wonderful benefits from exercise. Frequent and regular physical exercise boosts the immune system and helps prevent heart disease, cardiovascular disease, type 2 diabetes, and obesity. Exercise also improves mental health, helps prevent depression, helps to promote or maintain positive self-esteem, and can even augment an individual's sex appeal or body image, which is also found to be linked with higher levels of self esteem.

Not everyone benefits equally from exercise. There is tremendous variation in individual response to training. Most people will see a moderate increase in endurance from aerobic exercise, and some individuals will as much as double their oxygen uptake. As anyone begins to exercise regularly, they will start to see improvement by implementing a constant training routine.

Physiological Changes

Exercise creates several physiological and neuromuscular changes that will vary due to the type, frequency, duration, and intensity of the training regimen. If your training is meant for speed, you'll get faster. If you exercise in order to become stronger, you will get stronger. And if you train for endurance, you will be able to endure longer workouts. Genetics also play a significant role in how quickly and dramatically you are able to improve from your training. In order to see significant changes, it should take at least four to eight weeks. Once you stop your training, the beneficial changes that occurred will begin to disappear faster than they developed.

Heart Changes

The most important change that correlates with training occurs in the heart. During a workout, the heart pumps blood containing important oxygen, fluids, and nutrients to the muscles that are being worked. This increased blood flow drains the metabolic waste products away. The more blood pumped, the more oxygen is pumped to the heart and the better equipped the muscles become to extract the oxygen and use it to produce more work.

Heart Changes During Aerobic Exercise

The heart adapts during sustained aerobic exercise such as jogging, rowing, swimming, and cycling. These types of activities strengthen heart and lung function by increasing the blood pumped per stroke. A stroke is the amount of blood ejected with each heartbeat. In untrained people, exercise can increase the cardiac output from pumping 4-5 liters per minute at rest to 16-20 liters per minute during exercise.

Trained athletes, on the other hand, can increase up to eight times resting output, getting up to 40 liters per minute, which is brought about by training-induced increase in the stroke volume. A trained athlete's stroke volume increases 50 to 60 percent during exercise. This occurs due to an increase in the contraction force of the heart and a greater emptying of the heart chamber. The heart of an aerobically trained person increases in size primarily in the left ventricle, which pumps blood away from the heart to the working muscles.

Heart Changes in Strength Training

Strength training causes changes in the heart different from aerobic exercises. Your heart must generate more force with each beat to pump into blood vessels with increased pressure due to tightened muscles. This causes the wall of the left ventricle to thicken to increase the pressure. The thickened wall does not enlarge the internal chamber but can generate more force with each beat. Training for strength and aerobic exercise allows the heart to adapt proportionally to both types of exercise. Consistent training in both categories will result in easier workouts.

Changes to Circulatory System

When you are exercising, your blood flow is redistributed. The body sends less blood to the major organs, except the heart and brain, and more blood to muscles and skin. At rest, 20 percent of blood goes to the muscles compared to 88 percent at maximum exertion. Arteries and veins can constrict or dilate rapidly to redistribute blood flow to meet the body's needs. During exercise, arteries dilate in working muscles and blood flow increases causing many small vessels called capillaries to open allowing blood flow. Increased blood flow causes an increase in the exchange of oxygen, the release of heat, and the removal of metabolic waste like lactic acid and carbon dioxide. The nervous system secretes a hormone that tells the vessels to dilate in the heart and working muscles. With more training, this signal works more efficiently. The blood redistribution takes several minutes—suddenly starting or stopping exercise can cause you to be breathless, strain unprepared muscles or cause lightheadedness due to blood pooling in muscles. Blood flow through the capillaries is critical to maximum exertion. Through constant training over time, the number of capillaries in the working muscles increases. Also, blood becomes thinner to allow for the flow through the capillaries to occur more easily. During workouts, the number of red blood cells stays level, but more water and proteins are added to the plasma resulting in an increase in plasma volume and a decrease in the concentration of red blood cells. This is called dilution and is referred to as athlete's anemia.

Changes in Muscular System: Muscle oxygen consumption increases up to 70 times above resting values during exercise. More than 4,000 capillaries may deliver blood to each square millimeter of muscle. This enables more oxygen, hormones, and nutrients to be delivered to muscles improving their ability to produce work and store glycogen that provides energy. Strength training increases muscle size and strength, both of which develop more mitochondria, which uses oxygen to convert glucose to ATP. Different types of training affect the changes in your muscle fibers. There are two types of fibers: fast-twitch for speed and power and slow-twitch for endurance. Training does not increase fiber type, but it does maximize the fibers' abilities. Resistance training develops a greater contraction force and also increases the muscle fiber size up to 50 percent. Increase in muscle size comes from increased fiber size, not number. Men generally have bigger muscles than women due to more testosterone that develops muscle.

Disease of Energy

The Calorie

The international unit for energy is the joule. However, the more widely used term is the Calorie. This is important because when we refer to the term 'Calorie' we actually mean kilocalorie written as a capital C. A calorie—with a small c—is 1/1000 of a Calorie. In other words: 1 Calorie (C) = 1 Kilocalorie = 1000 calories (c). All food labels use an upper case C.

Obesity: Simply put, this is an excess proportion of total body fat. A person is considered obese when his or her weight is 20% or more above normal weight. Another common measure of obesity is the body mass index or BMI. A person is considered overweight if his or her BMI is between 25 and 30. A person is considered obese if his or her BMI is over 30. Morbid obesity is a term that means that a person is greater than 50% over normal weight, more than 100 pounds over normal weight, has a BMI of 40 or higher, or is sufficiently overweight to severely interfere with health or normal function. Obesity occurs when a person consumes more calories than he or she burns. For many people this boils down to eating too much and exercising too little. But there are other factors that also play a role in obesity.

- Age. As you get older, your body's ability to metabolize food slows down and you do not require as many calories to maintain your weight.
- Gender. Women tend to be more overweight than men. Men have a higher resting metabolic rate (meaning they burn more energy at rest) than women, so men require more calories to maintain their body weight.
- Physical activity. Active individuals require more calories than less active ones to maintain their weight. Additionally, physical activity tends to decrease appetite in obese individuals while increasing the body's ability to preferentially metabolize fat as an energy source.
- Psychological factors. Psychological factors also influence eating habits and obesity.

Obesity in the United States has been increasing in recent decades. Of all countries, the United States has the highest rate of obesity. In 1962, 13% of Americans were considered obese. In 2010, 35.7% of American adults were considered obese.

Diabetes is a common illness with a total of 8% of the population of the United States afflicted. It is a disease involving insulin, the hormone produced by the pancreas to control blood sugar. The role of insulin is to move glucose from the bloodstream into muscle, fat, and liver cells, where it can be used as fuel. People with diabetes have high blood sugar because either their pancreas does not make enough insulin or their cells do not respond to insulin normally. There are three types of diabetes.

Type 1 diabetes occurs when the body's own immune system destroys the insulin-producing cells of the pancreas (called beta cells). In people with type 1 diabetes, sugar isn't moved into the cells because insulin is not available. When sugar builds up in the blood instead of going into cells, the body's cells starve for nutrients and other systems in the body must provide energy for many important bodily functions.

Type 2 diabetes is the most common form of diabetes. Between 90% and 95% of the people with diabetes have Type 2 diabetes. Unlike those with type 1 diabetes, people with type 2 diabetes produce insulin. However, either their pancreas does not produce enough insulin or the body cannot use the insulin adequately. This is called insulin resistance. Type 2 diabetes tends to be related to genetics.

Gestational diabetes is a condition characterized by high blood sugar levels that is first recognized during pregnancy. The condition occurs in approximately 4% of all pregnancies.

Anorexia and Bulimia: Anorexia nervosa is an eating disorder that is now defined as a psychological disorder. The person with this has a distorted body image and an irrational fear of becoming overweight – so he or she deliberately attempts to lose weight. Even though the majority of patients are female, men can also suffer from anorexia nervosa. A person with anorexia nervosa weighs much less than he or she should - 15% or more below their ideal weight, has a BMI of 17.5 or less, has a preoccupation with body shape and weight, and has a severe fear of putting on weight. About 75% of reported anorexia nervosa onsets start between the ages 11-20. An exaggerated fear of losing control is mainly driven by low self-esteem and constant self-criticism. It is not uncommon for a patient to feel he or she has lost control after consuming a tiny amount of food.

Bulimia nervosa is also defined as a psychological disorder. The patient experiences regular bouts of serious overeating that are always followed by a feeling of guilt that can then lead to extreme reactions such as crash dieting, doing lots of exercise, and purging (deliberately vomiting). People with bulimia will eat much more than most people normally do and feel that they can't stop or control their eating. Unlike anorexia nervosa, bulimia nervosa is difficult to identify because the people who suffer from this disorder are not usually underweight. Because of the shame and guilt associated with the illness, patients are skilled in masking the symptoms. Long-term, the patient may experience malnutrition.

Questions – Chapter 1

1. Name the three types of foods that have nutritional value, provide energy, and act as building blocks for humans.
2. Explain the difference between monosaccharide and disaccharide.
3. What are the three steps of sugar metabolism ? What is the purpose/product of each step?
4. In your own words, explain what the oxygen debt is and how it can be advantageous.
5. What happens if the body has sufficient glucose and oxygen but is not exercising?
6. According to the chart in the chapter, what is your estimated BMR?
7. What are the three ways that heat is lost? (Provide a brief explanation of each)
8. What are some of the changes that occur in the body when exercising? Provide a brief description of each that you list.

CHAPTER 2:
The Lungs

Function of the Lungs

Sugar gives the body energy by providing it with electrons that are found in the food we eat. The body has trillions of 'engines' called mitochondria to extract this energy. In order to extract energy, it is necessary that the electrons have a target. This target is oxygen. Oxygen is the ultimate electron acceptor in the process called oxidation. As a result, our bodies need lots of oxygen. Conversely, the byproduct of energy production is carbon dioxide. Oxygen and carbon dioxide are carried around the body in the blood. The primary purpose of the lungs is to exchange these two gases by taking oxygen from the air we breathe and placing it into the blood while taking carbon dioxide from the blood and putting it back into the air. Our cells are always producing carbon dioxide. The more we exercise the more carbon dioxide is produced. In fact, it is the level of carbon dioxide in the blood that drives the breathing rate, not the lack of oxygen within the cells.

Most of the air that we breathe consists of the gas nitrogen – about 80 percent of it, in fact. Nitrogen is an inert gas that does not have any physiological function. About 20 percent of the air we breathe in is oxygen. The air we breathe out is quite different. All of the nitrogen comes out, but only about 16 percent of the oxygen comes out – having been used by the cells to produce energy. About four percent of the expired air is carbon dioxide, also a byproduct of energy production.

INSPIRATION		EXPIRATION
80%	Nitrogen	80%
20%	Oxygen	16%
0%	Carbon Dioxide	4%

The lungs do more than just exchange gases. First, they play a key role in keeping the pH, or acid level, of the body constant. This is incredibly important for proper function of muscles and organs. Carbon dioxide is acidic, and by expelling or retaining carbon dioxide, the lungs help maintain the proper acid level. They moisturize the air, which enable us to 'see' our breath in the winter. The lungs also help to maintain body temperature. This is particularly true in some animals that pant to expel hot air. Finally, the lungs play an important role in voice production.

Humans take a breath about 12-18 times per minute, usually subconsciously. When at rest, we breathe about six liters of air each minute. During exercise, our breathing rate increases to allow more oxygen to enter the blood and to remove carbon dioxide from the blood. When we stop exercising, our breathing rate returns to normal. The speed at which the breathing rate returns to normal after exercise is a good indicator of physical fitness.

Structure of the lungs

The lungs are divided into lobes. The right lung is divided into three lobes: the upper, middle, and lower lobes. However, the left lung is smaller and is only divided into two lobes. The left lung is slightly smaller to accommodate room for the heart, located below the left lung.

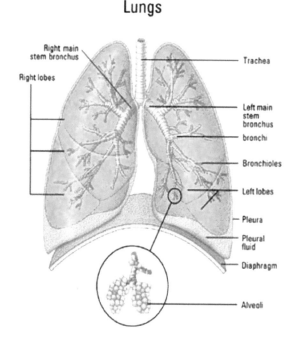

Lungs

When we breathe, air travels through the tracheobronchial tree. The tracheobronchial tree is a tubular system that leads into the lungs. It is sometimes simply called "the airway." Structural supporters called tracheal rings support the airway, keeping it from collapsing when we exhale or when there is an absence of air.

The airway begins with the mouth. The back of the mouth is called the pharynx. This extends down and becomes the trachea. The trachea then divides into the right and left bronchi. The two bronchi split into branches again. These branches act as paths for air to reach the bronchioles. These bronchioles then end where the very small air pouches known as alveoli are located. In all, there are sixteen splits from the trachea to alveolar sacs, making the tracheobronchial tree an extremely complex system.

The alveoli have extremely thin membranes that allow the passage of air directly into the lung tissue. When the lungs inflate and deflate, air passes in and out of the alveoli accordingly. Therefore, the alveoli are the reason that we are able to breathe.

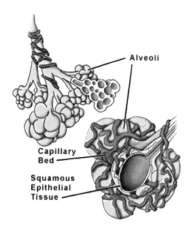

There are about 30 million alveoli in a newborn's lung. By about the age of eight years old, that number has increased to about 300 million at a rate of about 100,000 new alveoli per day. The number of alveoli does not increase after that. However, they do increase in diameter. This causes the total surface of the area of the lungs to be enormous. This convoluted surface has a total area of about 80 m^2, which is about half the size of a tennis court. This makes the lungs the organ that is most exposed to the environment and subject to many diseases.

Because the airway and lungs are so exposed to the environment, we breathe many things into our lungs each day including dust, smoke, bacteria, and viruses. The body has two ways of removing all of these objects. Large chunks are removed by coughing. Smaller particles are carried out by millions of small hairs called cilia. Cilia are tiny, just 0.1 mm long. They

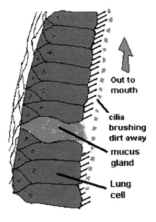

have a constant beating or wave-like motion that carries mucous and tiny dust particles up toward the mouth. Each cilium vibrates about 1,000 times per minute. The mucous moves at about one to two cm per minute. While this is not fast, it is efficient in removing unwanted particles from our lungs.

Some people have a genetic disease where they lack the bottom part of the cilia. As a result, they do not have the ability to remove particles or mucous from their lungs. This is called immotile ciliary syndrome. People with this syndrome are sick with pneumonia and other lung diseases quite a bit.

The alveoli are coated with pulmonary surfactant. The function of surfactant is to reduce the surface tension of the alveoli, enabling them to hold their shape. Therefore, surfactant is critically important to the proper function of the alveoli. The protection of the lungs, however, is left to the pleura. This is a thin membrane-like covering that surrounds the lungs. The main function of the pleura is to cushion and pad the lungs during respiration.

Taking a Breath

When we breath in, a series of events take place. First, the strong diaphragm muscles contract, causing them to drop into the abdomen. This increases the size of the chest cavity (the thorax). The enlarged volume drops the pressure in the thorax, causing the lungs to expand to fill that volume. As the lungs expand, the airways expand also, making the passageways where air travels much larger and, in turn, making it easier to take a breath. As the lungs expand, air moves through the airway, all the way to the alveoli, filling the enlarging lungs.

When we breathe out, the opposite happens. The diaphragm relaxes, and the thorax contracts and becomes smaller. The lungs in turn become smaller, forcing air back out through the airways and out of the mouth. At the same time, due to the increase in air pressure, the airways also try to collapse. If they were to collapse, of course, we could not breathe out. So, to prevent this from happening, two things occur. First, strong fibrous rings placed around the airway from the trachea to the alveoli prop the airway open. These are called tracheal rings and they protect the airway. The other way the airway is kept open is when we are forcing air out of our mouths, such as when we are exercising or blowing out a birthday candle. We will purse our lips together, causing backpressure on the airway helping it to stay open. In this manner, we can breathe out without the fear of our airways collapsing.

Breathing requires energy. In science this energy is called work. The harder we breathe, the more energy or work

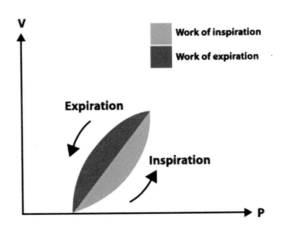

is required. In fact, as much as 90 percent of the body's energy is used in breathing. Looking at a pressure-volume curve of breathing, it is clear that the greater the volume that we inhale, the more pressure is required. The area in between these curves is a measure of the energy or the work needed for someone to breathe.

We breathe through our nostrils, not through our mouths. There are a number of reasons for this. First, air is moisturized in the chambers of the nose. This makes moving air through the passages easier. Occasionally we do breathe through our mouths, but this is usually reserved for when we exercise or when our nostrils are clogged up. Babies have not 'learned' how to breathe through their mouths. As a result, breathing can become difficult for a baby even with a mild cold.

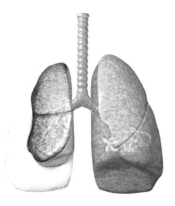

Because the thorax is usually at a lower pressure than the atmosphere, any hole that is created in the chest wall will cause air to move into the thorax. Such a hole can be created by any one of a number of events such as trauma from a broken rib, cutting a hole in the chest wall. A gunshot or knife wound can also do the same thing. When the chest wall is punctured, air rushes into the chest, causing pressure in the thorax to increase. This causes partial or total lung collapse. This condition is called a pneumo-thorax, meaning 'air in the chest.' It is often deadly. To correct this, a tube is inserted in to the space around the collapsed lung and then connected to a pump, literally sucking the air out of the thorax and re-expanding the lung.

Perfusion and Ventilation

The right side of the heart pumps the entire blood supply of the body into the lungs to exchange CO_2 for O_2. This process is called perfusion. The airway provides oxygen to the lungs, and this is called ventilation. The upper parts of the lungs (about five percent) are much better ventilated but have poor perfusion compared to the rest of the lungs. Conversely, the bottom part of the lungs (about five percent) are much better perfused but poorly ventilated. So these parts of the lungs do not work as well in gas exchange. The middle parts of the lungs (the remaining 90 percent) are both well-perfused and well-ventilated. This is where most of the exchanges of gases occur. When we exercise, more blood vessels form near the top of the lung and airways open at the bottom of the lungs, thus making the lungs more efficient in exchanging gasses.

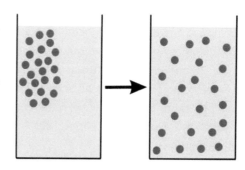

Air moves through the airways initially through the process of convection. This is the blowing or movement of air. You can feel the air move through your nostrils or mouth when you breathe. This is efficient and moves air all the way down to the opening of the alveoli. At this point, the expansion of the alveoli is complete and air motion stops. The oxygen must move to the end of the alveoli by the process called diffusion. This process is slow by comparison to con-vection. Once the oxygen molecule reaches the lining of the alveoli, it must then diffuse a second time across the lining of both the alveolar wall and the blood vessel wall. These two processes of diffusion take about three to four seconds to occur.

Hemoglobin

This is a very important molecule in the blood. It is found in the red blood cells. Its main purpose is to carry oxygen from the lungs to the organs and the rest of the body (such as muscles and other tissues) where it releases the oxygen to assist in extracting energy from the electrons found in the food. It helps to bring a little bit of the resultant carbon dioxide back to the lungs where it is expelled through the mouth.

The hemoglobin molecule is made up of four globular protein subunits, two alpha chains, and two beta chains. Each of the four subunits is bound to a structure called a heme group. At the center of the heme group is a ring of molecules called a porphyrin ring. At the center of the porphyrin ring is the important atom iron (Fe). This is where oxygen binds. Thus one molecule of hemoglobin can carry up to four oxygen molecules.

Oxygen does not mix with liquids (including blood) very well. (However, carbon dioxide mixes in liquids very well, which is why we have carbonated drinks rather than oxygenated drinks.) This is a real problem for moving oxygen around in blood. In fact, if the body had to depend on oxygen mixed in blood to carry oxygen to the cells, the heart would have to pump 140 liters per minute instead of four liters per minute. There needs to be a molecule to carry oxygen to the tissues and cells.

Oxygen does not bind to all four heme sites in hemoglobin simultaneously. Instead, once the first heme binds oxygen, it causes small changes in the structure of the corresponding proteins. These changes nudge the neighboring chains into a different shape, making them bind oxygen more easily. Thus, it is difficult to add the first oxygen molecule, but binding the second, third, and fourth oxygen molecules becomes progressively easier. This provides a great advantage as hemoglobin grabs onto oxygen. Each red blood cell can carry about one million molecules of oxygen.

Hemoglobin is 97 percent saturated with oxygen when it leaves the lungs and is about 75 percent saturated when it returns. When blood is in the lungs, where oxygen is plentiful, oxygen easily binds and fills up the hemoglobin molecule. Out in the muscles and tissues, the oxygen level is low and carbon dioxide level is high. At this point the hemoglobin releases its oxygen. As soon as the first oxygen molecule drops off, hemoglobin starts changing its shape. This prompts the remaining three oxygen molecules to be quickly released. In this way, hemoglobin picks up the largest possible load of oxygen in the lungs and delivers it quickly when needed out in the tissues.

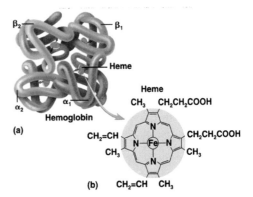

The mineral iron plays an important role in the body's delivery to and use of oxygen by working muscles. It binds oxygen to hemoglobin. The more oxygen there is being delivered, the greater the body's ability to perform work. For this reason, iron receives much attention for its role in supporting aerobic exercise. A lack of iron in the body can reduce the ability for endurance performance.

The Alveoli

The airways supply air to each lung; however, the airways continue to branch out and finally become millions of small sacs called alveoli. This is where the exchange of O_2 and CO_2 takes place. The alveoli are so very small – they are only 0.2 mm in diameter and the walls are a mere 0.4 micrometers thick – but they have a large surface area. They really look like and act like tiny interconnected balloons. The alveoli are lined with a type of fluid called surfactant, which is necessary to keep them functioning properly. Premature babies are at risk for being born without surfactant lining their alveoli, which causes a disease called respiratory distress syndrome that can be fatal to newborns.

Surface tension

This is a property caused by attraction of molecules and is responsible for many of the behaviors of liquids. It allows liquid to resist an external force. It is seen when objects (like a leaf or an insect) float on the surface of water, even though they are denser than water. It is important in the function of the lungs because it causes them to stick to the surface of the chest wall and prevents the collapse of the alveoli when we exhale.

The pressure inside of a balloon is inversely proportional to its radius. That is, the pressure increases as the radius is smaller. This is familiar to most people, as it is known to be more difficult to blow up a balloon when it is small and becomes easier as the balloon becomes bigger. The pressure inside of a balloon is also directly proportional to the surface tension. As surface tension increases, so does the pressure. All this can be shown in this equation:

$$Pressure = \frac{4 \; x \; surface \; tension}{radius}$$

A liquid with low-surface tension on its surface will also allow balloons to stay inflated longer than a balloon with a high-surface tension.

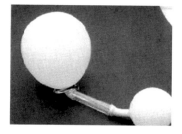

Let's say that two balloons are connected to each other with a tube. One of the balloons is bigger than the other, meaning it has a larger radius. Because the smaller balloon has a smaller radius, our equation states that it would have a larger internal pressure and would proceed to empty into the larger balloon until the pressures of the two balloons equalize. This is counter to what most people think would happen. But think about the last time you blew up a balloon. It was hard at first, but then became progressively easier as the balloon became larger. This is how it works for the alveoli. They are harder to inflate if they are completely empty, but easier to inflate as they get larger. This is why smaller alveoli want to collapse, and larger alveoli want to enlarge. This is not a good situation for keeping the lungs open and full of oxygen.

To prevent the collapse of alveoli, the inside of our alveoli are coated with surfactant, which changes the equation. Surfactant helps to keep smaller alveoli open. Surfactant in the lungs has a surface tension that changes. As the alveoli get smaller, the surface tension also gets smaller. In fact, at about one-fourth its maximum size, an alveoli's surface tension is decreasing so rapidly that pressure inside also drops. This keeps the alveoli about one-fourth of the way full, which in turn allows for easier re-inflation when we take in a breath. Because of the surfactant, the alveoli are not allowed to empty completely. That means that lungs retain some air when exhalation ends. This makes it much easier to inhale. For infants and others where surfactant is absent, the alveoli completely collapse and require a large pressure to reopen them. Small infants sometimes aren't strong enough to generate the pressure needed to reopen the alveoli and can suffocate.

It is essential for survival that our alveoli do not completely empty at the end of an exhalation. It simply would require too much work to reopen them. Thankfully, the changing surface tension of surfactant keeps the alveoli at least partially full at the end of exhalation. However, there are some conditions where some of the alveoli will collapse anyway. Most everyone will occasionally take deep breaths or sighs without being aware of it. This is to reopen any collapsed alveoli. Also, in a chest injury where it hurts to take a deep breath, alveoli can collapse and be very dangerous if not treated right away. This is called atelectasis. Sometimes it is necessary to force large amounts of air into the patient's lungs occasionally to reopen collapsed alveoli.

Diseases of the Lung and Airway

The air we breathe is often filled with contaminants, harmful bacteria, viruses, allergens, and hazardous cancer-causing chemicals. There are too many airway and lung illnesses to cover, but there are a few common ones that most people either have had or know someone who has had them.

Pneumonia

This is an infection within the lungs that is caused by bacteria, viruses, fungi, or parasites. It is characterized primarily by inflammation of the alveoli in the lungs or by alveoli that are filled with fluid. A very serious condition, pneumonia can make a person very sick or even cause death. Although the disease can occur in young and healthy people, it is most dangerous for older adults, babies, and people with other diseases or impaired immune systems. Most people with pneumonia recover, but about five percent will succumb to the condition.

Asthma

This is a chronic lung disease that inflames and narrows the airways. Asthma causes recurring episodes of wheezing, chest tightness, shortness of breath, and sometimes coughing. In the United States, more than 25 million people are known to have asthma, about seven million of whom are children. People with asthma tend to react strongly to certain inhaled substances such as pollen or animal dander. When the airways react, the muscles around them tighten. This narrows the airways, causing less air to flow into the lungs. Sometimes asthma symptoms are mild and go away on their own or after minimal treatment with asthma medicine that opens the airways. When symptoms are more serious, hospitalization is necessary. Inhaling medicines that open the airways treats it.

Common Cold

The common cold is a viral infection of the upper respiratory tract — the nose and throat. A common cold is usually harmless, although it may not feel that way. If it's not a runny nose, sore throat, and cough, it's the watery eyes, sneezing, and congestion — or maybe all of the above. In fact, because any one of more than 100 viruses can cause a common cold, signs and symptoms tend to vary greatly. There is no cure but thankfully they usually only last for a few days.

Bronchitis

When the lining of the bronchial tubes becomes inflamed or infected, the condition is called bronchitis. Bronchitis reduces the amount of air and oxygen that can flow into the lungs and causes heavy mucus to form in the airways. Bronchitis is considered to be either acute or chronic. Acute bronchitis is a shorter illness that usually lasts from few days to a week and is commonly caused by a viral infection. In addition to viruses, bacteria, exposure to tobacco smoke, exposure to pollutants, or even acid from the stomach (caused by gastro-esophageal reflux disease or GERD) can also cause acute bronchitis. Chronic bronchitis is characterized by a persistent, mucus-producing cough on most days of the month for most of the year. Cigarette smoking usually causes chronic bronchitis.

COPD

Chronic Obstructive Pulmonary Disease is characterized by destruction of the alveoli. Cigarette smoking is the most common cause of COPD. Breathing in other kinds of irritants such as pollution, dust, or chemicals, may also cause or contribute to COPD. However, smoking is the main cause. It makes it hard for people to breathe. Chronic bronchitis and emphysema are common COPDs. Treatment can make you more comfortable, but there is no cure.

Lung cancer

This is the uncontrolled growth of abnormal cells that start off in one or both lungs. Smoking almost always causes lung cancer. Being exposed to cigarette smoke causes lung cancer as well. As tumors become larger and more numerous, they undermine the lung's ability to provide the bloodstream with oxygen. According to the National Cancer Institute, there were about 227,000 new lung cancer diagnoses and 160,400 lung-cancer related deaths in the USA in 2012. Lung cancer is by far the number one cancer killer. The American Cancer Society says that lung cancer makes up 14 percent of all newly diagnosed cancers in the USA today. Furthermore, annually more patients die from lung cancer alone than prostate, breast, and colon cancers combined.

Chapter 2 – Questions

1. What percentage of the oxygen inhaled is retained and used in the body?
2. What function, aside from gas exchange, do the lungs have and why is this function so important?
3. Describe the structure of the lungs.
4. Describe the structure of the airway.
5. What are the two ways in which the body removes debris from the airway?
6. Why is surfactant so important?
7. Explain the process that occurs when we take a breath.
8. What are some of the diseases of the lungs? Describe the symptoms of each disease you list.

CHAPTER 3:
The Heart

The supply of oxygen and glucose is so important to the body that the heart is the first major organ to develop in the embryo. Just eight weeks after conception the heart is working to circulate blood to the tissues of the fetus. We have learned that the cells of the body act like individual engines. In order for them to function, they must have food to supply electrons and oxygen from the air to release energy and a way to dispose of carbon dioxide and heat. Since the body has about a trillion cells, an elaborate transportation system is needed.

Heart and blood facts

On average, the heart beats about 100,000 times per day. That's three billion times in a lifetime.
About eight million red blood cells die every second, and that same number is born every second.
There are valves in all the veins of the body (not the arteries) to make sure blood blows in one direction.
When it is beating, the heart is about as firm as a tennis ball.
It takes about 20 seconds for one red blood cell to travel through the entire circulatory system.

Circulation within the Heart

The heart is basically a double pump. It provides the force needed to circulate the blood through the two major circulatory systems: the pulmonary circulation in the lungs and the systemic circulation in the rest of the body. Blood circulates through one system before being pumped by the heart to the second system. The heart is split into four cavities. The two top chambers are called the right and left atria, and the bottom chambers are the right and left ventricles. They are separated by valves, which allow for blood to be pumped into the next cavity while preventing backflow into the previous one. If the valves become diseased, the flow of blood becomes disrupted. In some cases these valves can be replaced surgically.

Deoxygenated blood enters the superior and inferior vena cava from the body. From there it travels into the right atrium and then through the tricuspid valve into the right ventricle. From the right ventricle, blood is pumped through the pulmonary valve and into the pulmonary artery where it is taken to the lungs. In the lungs, the deoxygenated red blood cells are given oxygen and then pumped back into the heart through the pulmonary veins. These veins place the blood into the left atrium where it quickly moves through the mitral valve to the left ventricle. The left ventricle provides the contracting force that pumps the blood through the aortic valve, into the aorta, and to the rest of the body. The blood travels through even smaller arterioles and then smaller capillaries. Once the cells remove the oxygen, the deoxygenated blood flows back to the heart through the veins.

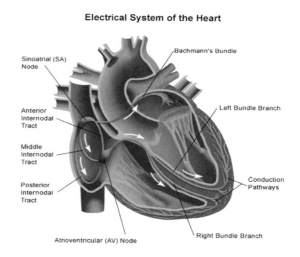

Electrical System of the Heart

Arteries always carry oxygenated blood away from the heart, and veins always carry deoxygenated blood to the heart. There are only two exceptions to this rule and both occur in the heart. The pulmonary artery carries deoxygenated blood from the heart to the lungs. It is called an artery because it's taking the blood away from the heart. The other exception is the pulmonary veins, which carry oxygenated blood from the lungs into the left atrium. Since blood is going into the heart it is called a vein.

mmHg

This stands for millimeters mercury. It is a common unit of pressure in the body. It states how high the heart could pump mercury vertically into the air.

The blood pressure as it leaves the heart is normally about 125 mmHg. However, the blood pressure as it reenters the heart is about zero. Almost the entire pressure drop occurs across the arterioles and the capillary bed of the circulatory system. This means that the heart is a pump that raises the pressure from 0 to 125 mmHg. When the right atrium beats, the blood pressure is about 5 mmHg. The right ventricle pumps with a pressure of about 25 mmHg. When blood returns to the left atrium, it will contract with about 8 mmHg. The left ventricle pumps with about 125 mmHg and the cycle has started all over again.

	Pressure
Right atrium	5 mmHg
Right ventricle	25 mmHg
Left atrium	8 mmHg
Left ventricle	125 mmHg

Blood

The blood volume is not uniformly divided between the pulmonary and systemic circulations. At any one time about 80 percent of the blood is in the systemic circulation and about 20 percent is in the lungs. Of the blood in the systemic circulation, about 25 percent is in the arteries and capillaries, and 75 percent is in the veins. That means that the veins hold a significant amount of blood. They are in fact the 'storage' areas for our blood.

While we normally think of blood as bright red, most of the blood in the body is dark red. The venous blood is depleted of the oxygen that makes the blood bright red so it appears dark red, with a bluish color. Blood appears to be a red liquid slightly thicker than water. That is because about 55 – 60 percent of our blood is composed of plasma, which is a nearly clear fluid like water. Plasma is composed of clotting factors and immunoglobulins that help to fight infection. About 40 – 45 percent of our blood is made of red blood cells. (That percentage is called the hematocrit, a common lab value in medicine.) The red cells develop in the bone marrow and circulate for about 100–120 days until they 'die.' About one percent of our blood is made up of white blood cells that fight infection. The blood also contains platelets that are important in clotting. Platelets live only three days. This means that about five million platelets die each second and an equal number are produced. The blood also acts as a transport mechanism for small amounts of hormones that control chemical processes in the body. Certain electrolytes (potassium, sodium and calcium) are also found in the blood and are crucial to the proper functioning of the body.

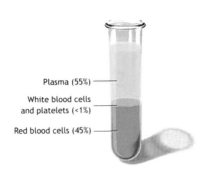

Plasma (55%)

White blood cells and platelets (<1%)

Red blood cells (45%)

Other Functions of Blood

Although we have emphasized the role of blood in gas exchange, an equally important function of the blood is to carry the body's liquid wastes to the kidneys. By filtration of the blood, the kidneys keep the makeup of the blood very constant despite large fluctuations in our diet. The kidneys are well vascularized in order to filter the blood. Normally 1 to 1.5 liters of blood flow through the kidneys each minute.

The blood also plays an important role in distributing and dissipating heat in the body. The venous blood returning from the limbs can be routed close to the skin to increase heat losses in warm weather. Conversely, in cold weather venous blood can be routed internally close to the artery carrying blood to the limb. This way, the cool venous blood takes up some of the heat from the warm arterial blood and carries it back to the heart. This counter-current principle lowers heat losses from the extremities and skin in cold weather.

How quickly does the blood flow?

As the blood moves away from the heart, the arteries branch and re-branch many times to carry blood to the various tissues. The smallest blood vessels are the capillaries. There are millions of them in the body.

As the blood goes from the aorta into the smaller arteries and arterioles with greater total cross-sectional areas, the velocity of the blood decreases just as the velocity of a river decreases at a wide portion. The average velocity in the aorta is about 300mm/s, and that in a capillary is only about 1mm/s. It is in the capillaries that the exchange of oxygen and carbon dioxide takes place, and this low velocity allows time for diffusion of the gases to occur.

The Cardiac Cycle

Because of its role in supplying blood to the entire body, the left ventricle is of great importance. It begins to fill up with blood when the mitral valve opens. About 90 – 95 percent of the blood in the left atrium flows into the left ventricle without the need for the left atrium to contract. This is represented by point A on the chart. The volume in the left ventricle increases as blood continues to enter. The line between point A and B on the chart represents this. Then a trigger from the brain signals the left ventricle to start to contract or begin systole. The contraction immediately causes the mitral valve to close making a sound – which we often say as 'lub' in the 'lub – dub' of heart sounds. This is point B on the chart.

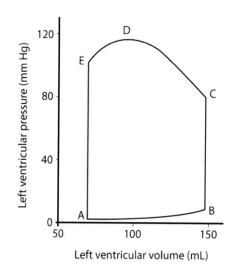

However, even though the heart muscle is squeezing, the blood cannot leave the left ventricle because not only is the mitral valve closed, but the aortic valve is closed also. There is not enough pressure to open it up. So while the ventricle muscle is tightening, it does not change its size. This is analogous to someone grabbing a doorknob and squeezing tightly; it will not change its shape. In its effort to push blood out, the left ventricle will continue to squeeze until there is enough pressure to open the aortic valve and eject blood. The line between point B and C on the chart represents this. This aortic valve opens about 0.1 second after systole began and the mitral valve had closed. The pressure needed to open up the aortic valve is called the diastolic blood pressure and is the bottom number when you take your blood pressure. It is usually about 70 – 80 mmHg in most people. This is point C on the chart.

So why didn't the aortic valve open as soon as the left ventricle began to contract? This is an important question as the answer affects our health. There are factors that keep the aortic valve from opening immediately. These are things such as how sticky blood might be, the weight of the blood, frictional forces, and narrow arteries. All of these make it difficult for the muscle of the left ventricle to push blood into the circulation and are collectively called system vascular resistance.

Once the aortic valve opens, blood is quickly ejected from the left ventricle. This is the line from point C to point E. When the pressure in the ventricle falls below the pressure in the aorta, the aortic valve will close. This is at point E. However, the line from C and E is not a straight line. The left ventricle continues to generate pressure so that it can get blood to the brain and other parts of the body. This maximum pressure is called the systolic blood pressure and is the upper number when you get your blood pressure taken. This is point E on the chart.

Finally, when the aortic valve closes at point D, the pressure in the left ventricle falls precipitously until the mitral valve opens again at point A and the cycle beings again. The line between point E and A on the chart represents this. The area within the loop defines the energy needed by the ventricle during one cardiac cycle.

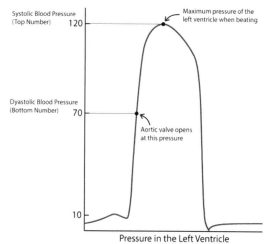

Blood Pressure

Remember, the heart is essentially a series of pumps, and pumps create pressure. The left ventricle is the strongest of the 4 pumps in the heart. The pressure needed to open the aortic valve and eject blood is called the diastolic blood pressure. The maximum pressure created by the heart is called the systolic blood pressure. If the systolic blood pressure becomes too high, blood pressure in the arteries around the whole body also becomes high. This can cause them to burst and bleed. When this occurs in the brain it is called a stroke. If it happens in the eye, it can cause blindness. If it happens in the kidneys, it can cause kidney failure. If it happens in a blood vessel in the chest or abdomen, it is called an aneurysm. Then if the diastolic blood pressure is too high, it means that the heart has to work harder to get blood out of the left ventricle. The higher the diastolic blood pressure the more difficult it becomes. If it gets too high, then blood does not leave the ventricle very well. This is one of the causes of heart failure and is the leading cause of death in the United States. This is usually caused by vessels being too constricted or by having too much blood in the arteries.

	Definition	Normal	Diseases
Systolic Blood Pressure	The maximum pressure created by the left ventricle when it beats (systole)	100 – 120 mmHg	Stroke, blindness, kidney failure, heart disease, aneurysm
Diastolic Blood Pressure	The pressure necessary for the left ventricle to open up the aortic valve and eject blood	60 – 80 mmHg	Heart failure

Measuring Blood Pressure

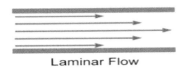

Laminar Flow

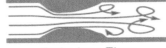

Turbulent Flow

Blood flow in the body is generally smooth flow (called laminar flow) and is hard to detect. This type of flow is similar to that of a slow, wide river moving along without making a sound. However, similar to rapids in a river, under certain conditions this smooth flow of blood can be disrupted and become turbulent. This fact is used to measure blood pressure because turbulence generates sound waves that can be heard with a stethoscope.

The smooth flow that normally occurs in the arteries produces little vibration of the arterial wall and therefore produces no sounds. However, when an artery is partially constricted, blood flow becomes turbulent causing the artery to vibrate and produce sounds. When measuring blood pressure, turbulent flow will occur when the cuff pressure is greater than the diastolic pressure and less than the systolic blood pressure. Initially the cuff is inflated to a level higher than the systolic blood pressure. Thus the artery is completely compressed, so there is no blood flow and no sounds are heard. The pressure is slowly decreased. At the point where the systolic pressure exceeds the cuff pressure, the sounds are first heard as blood passes in turbulent flow in the partially constricted artery. Sounds will continue to be heard as the cuff pressure is further lowered. However, when the cuff pressure reaches the diastolic pressure, the sounds disappear as the blood pressure is greater than the cuff pressure and the artery returns to being fully open, thus making no sounds.

Pulses

There are two pulses in the human body. The first is the well-known common arterial pulse. It is the one that most people feel in their wrists. The second is not as well known and is called the jugular pulse and is seen in the jugular vein in the neck.

In order to create the arterial pulse, blood is forced into the aorta during systole that not only moves the blood, but also sets up a pressure wave that travels through the arteries. The pressure wave expands the arterial walls as it travels, and you can feel this as the pulse. The speed at which the pulse travels is much faster than the blood. It is about 4 m/s in the aorta, 8 m/s in the large arteries, and 16 m/s in the small arteries of young adults. Consequently, the pulse is felt in the radial artery at the wrist about 0.1 seconds after blood leaves the heart into the aorta. With advancing age, the arteries become more rigid and the pulse wave moves even faster.

Blood Circulation in a Developing Baby

During pregnancy, the circulation of blood in the developing baby is different than in an adult. The fetus is connected by the umbilical cord to the placenta, the organ that develops and implants in the mother's uterus during pregnancy. The fetus receives all the necessary nutrition, oxygen, and life support from the mother through the placenta. Waste products and carbon dioxide from the fetus are sent back through the umbilical cord and placenta to the mother's circulation to be eliminated.

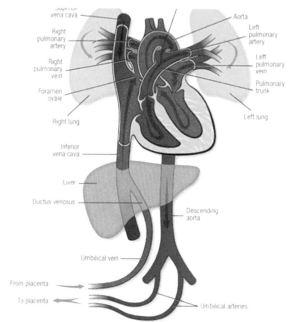

The fetal circulatory system uses shunts to bypass certain body parts – in particular, the lungs and liver – that are not fully developed while the fetus is still in the womb. The shunts that bypass the lungs are called the foramen ovale, which move blood from the right atrium of the heart to the left atrium, and the ductus arteriosus, which moves blood from the pulmonary artery to the aorta.

Oxygen and nutrients from the mother's blood are transferred across the liver into the inferior vena cava, a major vein connected to the heart. This shunt is called the ductus venosus. A small amount of blood goes directly to the liver to give it the oxygen and nutrients it needs.

In the fetal heart, the blood takes a different pathway than it does in a matured heart. Blood enters the right atrium, the chamber on the upper right side of the heart. When the blood enters the right atrium, most of it flows through the foramen ovale into the left atrium. Blood then passes into the left ventricle and then to the aorta.

In the fetus, the placenta does the work of breathing instead of the lungs. As a result, only a small amount of the blood continues on to the lungs. Most of this blood is bypassed or shunted away from the lungs through the ductus arteriosus to the aorta. Most of the circulation to the lower body is supplied by blood passing through the ductus arteriosus.

This blood then enters the umbilical arteries and flows into the placenta. In the placenta, carbon dioxide and waste products are released into the mother's circulatory system, and oxygen and nutrients from the mother's blood are released into the fetus's blood.

At birth, the umbilical cord is clamped and the baby no longer receives oxygen and nutrients from the mother. With the first breaths of life, the lungs begin to expand. As the lungs expand, the alveoli in the lungs are cleared of fluid. An increase in the baby's blood pressure and a significant reduction in blood pressure in the lungs reduce the need for the ductus arteriosus to shunt blood. These changes promote the closure of the shunt. In addition, the pressure in the left atrium of the heart increases, which decreases the pressure in the right atrium. The shift in pressure stimulates the foramen ovale to close. The closure of the ductus arteriosus and foramen ovale completes the transition of fetal circulation to newborn circulation.

Diseases of the Heart and Circulatory System

Coronary Artery Disease and Heart Attack: If blood flow to the heart is impaired, oxygen delivery to the heart muscle drops rapidly, while the concentration of waste products such as carbon dioxide increases. If this occurs in any tissue, it is known as ischemia. The arteries that take oxygenated blood to the heart muscle are called the coronary arteries. Over years, cholesterol plaques can build up within the coronary arteries, causing them to narrow gradually. When the coronary arteries are occluded, the patient may experience chest pain, known as angina. If heart muscle suffers irreversible damage it is classified as myocardial infarction, or heart attack.

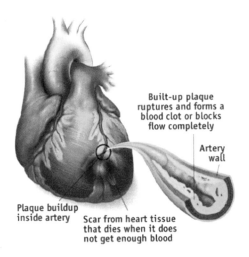

Built-up plaque ruptures and forms a blood clot or blocks flow completely

Artery wall

Plaque buildup inside artery

Scar from heart tissue that dies when it does not get enough blood

Heart Failure: When the pumping function of the heart fails or becomes impaired, fluid collects in the lungs and other tissues, leading to congestion. Heart failure can be the end result of any cardiac disease that impairs the heart's ability to pump blood, including poor valve function, high diastolic blood pressure, heart attack, or even infection. Heart failure causes fluid to accumulate in the lungs. Patients suffering from heart failure experience a variety of symptoms including shortness of breath, chest pain or tightness, fatigue, inability to sleep, increased nighttime urination, swelling of the lower limbs, and abdominal pain. All of these symptoms are a result of insufficient circulation throughout the body.

Valvular Diseases: Bad heart valves can be classified as being either stenotic (narrow) or regurgitant (leaky). Either condition can cause turbulent blood flow within the heart or the large vessels, which can lead to further damage. A stenotic valve obstructs flow, while a regurgitant valve allows flow in the wrong direction. Both conditions result in heart failure if left untreated. Bad heart valves can be replaced surgically if needed.

Peripheral Vascular Disease: This is a disease in which blood vessels become restricted or blocked in the arms or the legs. Typically, the patient has peripheral vascular disease from atherosclerosis. Atherosclerosis is a disease in which fatty plaques form in the inside walls of blood vessels. Both veins and arteries may be affected, but the disease is usually arterial. All the symptoms and consequences of peripheral vascular disease are related to restricted blood flow. There are many causes of peripheral vascular disease. One major risk factor is smoking cigarettes. Since peripheral vascular disease is seen mainly in the legs, these sensations usually occur when walking. Quitting smoking and implementing medicine, a better diet, and exercise are all methods to treat this disease.

Aneurysm: an aneurysm is an enlargement of part of the aorta that extends through the abdominal area and at times, the upper portion of the aorta in the chest. The aorta is the main blood vessel that carries blood from the heart to the rest of the body. Like most arteries, the aorta is elastic, which allows it to be filled with blood under high pressure. An aneurysm develops when the wall of the artery becomes weakened and distended like a balloon. A bubble in a garden hose would be an appropriate comparison to illustrate an aneurysm. Aneurysms usually are discovered before they produce symptoms, such as back pain, but like a weakened garden hose, they may rupture if they become too large. Since a ruptured aneurysm is extremely dangerous and can cause life-threatening bleeding, aneurysms are best corrected by an operation before this happens. People who are at risk are those over at 60. Other factors are family history, smoking, and inherited weakness in the blood vessel wall, high blood pressure, and high cholesterol.

Capillaries and Angiogenesis

The vascular system of the human body is composed of approximately 60,000 miles of blood vessels, enough vessels to circle the earth nearly two and a half times. These vessels form an incredible network, branching throughout the body to supply different tissues with oxygen and energy. Blood begins its path in the heart, exiting through a large valve and passing into the aorta. From there, it branches further into continually smaller branches. The smallest form of a blood vessel is known as a capillary.

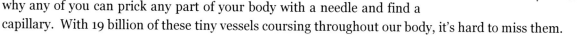

What is a capillary? Capillaries are small tubes measuring from 8 to 12 μm. This is small enough to force red blood cells to pass through in single file. The small nature of capillaries allows for oxygen molecules to pass through them and supply tissue with oxygen in a process known as diffusion. Every tissue in our body needs a blood supply, which explains why any of you can prick any part of your body with a needle and find a capillary. With 19 billion of these tiny vessels coursing throughout our body, it's hard to miss them.

What is angiogenesis? Blood vessels form in a process known as angiogenesis, from the Greek angeion, meaning "vessel", and genesis, meaning "origin or creation." This vessel formation supplies all the tissue in our body with blood. It does not occur normally in adults other than to heal wounds and in the monthly menstrual cycle in women. One exception arises in cancerous tumors. Tumors can grow without a blood supply to about 0.5 mm3, or about the size of the tip of a ballpoint pen.

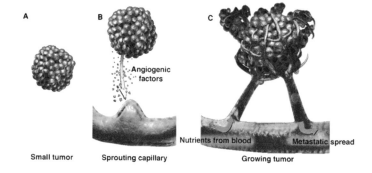

These tumors are very common, growing in nearly all of our thyroids by age 70, but without a blood supply they are harmless and cannot metastasize. When a tumor induces angiogenesis through secretion of various growth factors, it can then expand with the nutrients it receives from its newly found blood supply. Through this same network of newly formed capillaries, it can metastasize and seek other parts of the body to pollute.

Cancer in many ways parallels an embryo. They both require a supply of nutrients from a host. After meiosis occurs in a fertilized ovum, the embryonic cells begin to divide rapidly and migrate, forming complex organs through different clusters of cells, eventually forming a living organism. Cancer cells also have this ability to divide and migrate. It is becoming apparent that the most important mechanism in the metastasis of a cancer cell is its ability to resurrect the qualities that it once had in its embryonic stages. So, in a sense, a cell afflicted with cancer is not breaking down after years of service, but returning to its juvenile state. It is worthwhile to look for relatively harmless ways to kill these rogue cells. Diet in and of itself can play an important role in this counterattack.

How can we inhibit angiogenesis in tumors? Could it be the frequent consumption of soybeans in Japan that gives their country the highest life expectancy in the world? Do Sudanese and Syrian diets coincide with their low cancer rates? It has been shown that antiangiogenic factors found in certain foods can diminish the rate of angiogenesis in tumors. Foods like strawberries, soy beans, artichokes, dark chocolate, olive oil, and many others provide a natural supply of angiogenic inhibitors to battle the spread of cancer.

One in four men and one in five women in the US have the risk of dying from cancer. Vast amounts of money are spent each year to further the research on cancer treatment and prevention. One of these methods is simply learning to eat the right foods in order to starve cancerous tumors of their blood supply.

Chapter 3 – Questions

1. Discuss the flow of blood through the heart.
2. What is the role of arteries? What is the role of veins? What are the two exceptions to the general roles of arteries and veins?
3. Briefly describe the composition of blood.
4. What are the functions that blood performs in the body?
5. What are the normal systolic and diastolic blood pressures? What happens if these pressures become too high?
6. Why do fetal hearts have shunts?
7. What are some of the diseases of the heart or circulatory system? Describe some of the symptoms of each disease that you list.
8. What role does angiogenesis play in the growth of tumors?

CHAPTER 4:

The Eye

Vision

The eyes are the organs by which we are able to see the world around us. Although we perform this action every waking minute of our lives, the process by which it is achieved is very complicated. The keystone to vision is light. When one looks at an object, the light reflected off that object is what ends up being passed through the eye and eventually perceived by the brain as an image. In order to understand how light goes from the opening of the eye to being transformed into a signal in the brain, we must begin with the anatomy of the eye itself.

Light reflects off an object and enters the eye. The first thing light touches when entering the eye is a thin veil of tears that coats the front of the eye. Behind this lubricating moisture is the front window of the eye, called the cornea. This clear covering helps to focus the light (in fact, most of the focusing occurs at this surface). On the other side of the cornea is more moisture. This clear, watery fluid is called the aqueous humor, and it circulates throughout the front part of the eye (anterior chamber in the image below), keeping a constant pressure within the eye.

After light passes through the aqueous humor, it passes through the pupil. This is the central circular opening in the colored part of the eye—also called the iris. Depending on how much light there is, the iris may contract or dilate, respectively limiting or

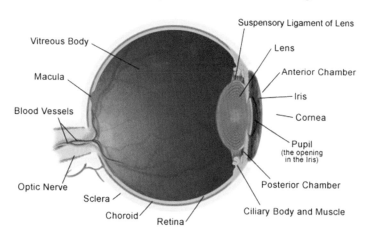

increasing the amount of light that travels deeper into the eye. The light then goes through the lens, which, just like the lens of a camera, also focuses the light. This is the variable focus of the eye. It does not focus the light as much as the cornea but the lens changes shape to focus light on the back of the eye.

This focused light now beams through the center of the eye. Again the light is bathed in moisture, this time in a clear jelly known as the vitreous. Surrounding the vitreous is the retina. Light reaches its final destination in the photoreceptors of the retina. The retina is the inner lining of the back of the eye. It's like a movie screen or the film of a camera. The focused light is projected onto its flat, smooth surface. However, unlike a movie screen, the retina has many working parts. Here are a few of the important parts:

- **Blood vessels.** Blood vessels within the retina bring nutrients to the retina's nerve cells.
- **Macula.** This is the bull's-eye at the center of the retina. The dead center of this bull's-eye is called the fovea. Because it's at the focal point of the eye, it has more of the specialized light-sensitive nerve endings (called photoreceptors) than any other part of the retina.
- **Photoreceptors.** There are two kinds of photoreceptors: rods and cones. These specialized nerve endings convert the light into electro-chemical signals. The rods help us see in the dark, differentiating between light and dark. The cones allow us to see colors; there are different cones for different colors.
- **Sclera.** This is the tough, fibrous, and white outside wall of the eye connected to the clear cornea in front. It protects the delicate structures inside the eye. Normally, light does not reach this layer.

Signals sent from the photoreceptors travel along nerve fibers to a nerve bundle that exits the back of the eye. This bundle is collectively called the optic nerve, which sends the signals to the visual center in the back of the brain.

Function of the lens

The lens is a transparent structure that allows the eye to adapt for both near and distant vision. Its transparency allows for light to pass through freely. It is also circular and biconvex, meaning that both sides bulge outwards similar to a magnifying glass. These characteristics allow the lens sufficient flexibility to perform its two primary functions: refraction and accommodation. Refraction is the bending of light and it occurs when the lens, along with the cornea, bends light rays in order to focus them onto the retina. Accommodation is an adjustment of the eye that permits focus on objects both near and far. This adjustment is achieved by changes in the shape of the lens controlled by the muscles on the edge of the lens called the cilliary muscle.

The ciliary muscle is a circular ring of smooth muscle that resides behind the iris and is attached to small fibers that suspend the lens. When viewing a near object, the ciliary muscle contracts, which leads to relaxation of the surface of the lens to make it more curved. The increase in curvature further bends the light rays onto the retina, focusing its view.

Conversely, in order to view an object that is far away, the ciliary muscle relaxes, causing the suspensory fibers to tighten, effectively flattening the lens. The flattened lens weakly refracts the light onto the back surface of the retina, allowing for focus on the distant object.

The lens and the cornea are the two major components that focus the light beam on the retina. The cornea is responsible for about 70 percent of the refractive power while the lens only accounts for about 30 percent. The lens is responsible for focusing the image on the surface of the retina. Most vision problems are *refractive problems*. A refractive problem occurs when the focal point of the image formed by the cornea and lens is not at the same place as the retina.

- Farsightedness (hyperopia) is a condition in which an image of a distant object becomes focused behind the retina, making objects up close appear out of focus.

- Nearsightedness (myopia) is a condition in which an image of a distant object becomes focused in front of the retina, making distant objects appear out of focus. Myopia is the most common lens error seen in children and can be corrected with eyeglasses or contact lenses.
- Astigmatism is a condition in which an abnormal curvature of the cornea can cause two focal points to fall in two different locations, making objects up close and at a distance appear blurry.

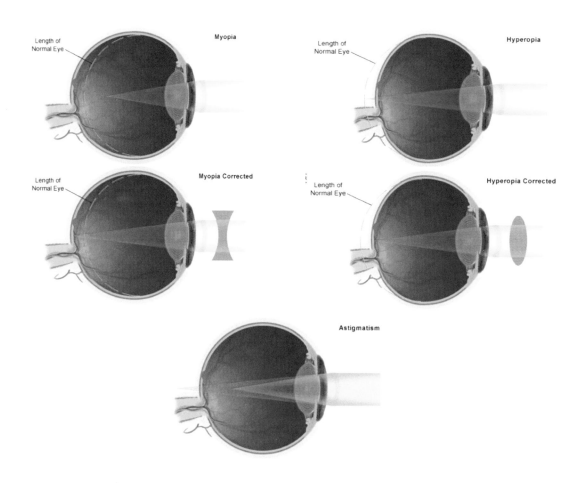

Diseases of the eye

Blindness: This is either a complete absence of vision or marked limitation of the visual fields. Legal blindness is a visual acuity of 20/200 or less after correction with lenses or glasses. Although there are many different causes of blindness, in general terms, anything that impedes light from reaching the back of the eye or interrupts nerve impulses transmitted from the optic nerve to the brain will impair vision. Blindness may occur in the following circumstances: light is not reaching the retina for a variety of reasons, the retina itself is damaged, nerve impulses are not transferred to the brain appropriately as a result of a disorder of the optic nerve, or the brain's visual cortex is damaged.

Macular degeneration: This is a major cause of gradual, painless, bilateral central vision loss in the elderly occurring in more than 10 million people in the United States. The macula is the central, 'bull's eye,' part of the retina onto which light reflected off an object is projected and converted by photoreceptors into impulses. Macular degeneration occurs when the macula itself gradually begins to fail. This occurs in two types: "dry" and "wet." The dry form, occurring in 80-90 percent of cases, involves the thinning of the macula as its cells gradually disappear over time. People with macular degeneration usually become legally blind. However, many are still able to perform daily tasks even with decreased central vision. At the moment there is no cure for this disorder, but controlling blood pressure and changing diet to include more antioxidants may help prevent the disease from worsening. Wearing sunglasses to protect the macula and eating a diet rich in a variety of fruits and vegetables can also prevent it.

Glaucoma: This is the third leading cause of blindness worldwide and second leading cause of blindness in the United States. In a normal eye, fluid in the front of the eye drains into drainage canals collectively called the trabecular meshwork. Glaucoma can be thought of as a clogged drain within this pathway. It occurs when the fluid within the eye reaches unhealthy levels due to clogged drainage canals, leading to increased eye pressure and eventual damage to the optic nerve.

If left untreated, glaucoma can lead to complete vision loss. Fortunately, there are multiple treatment options for those with glaucoma. Medications and eye drops are available that reduce pressure within the eye by either improving drainage of fluid or decreasing the amount of fluid produced within the eye. Laser surgery may also be performed in order to enlarge drainage pathways.

Cataracts: This is a clouding of the lens that causes gradual, painless, blurred vision. They are the number one cause of blindness worldwide. By age 80, more than half of all people in the United States will either have a cataract or will have had one removed. Although some cataracts can be congenital (occurring at birth or shortly thereafter), the majority of cataracts occur with aging.

Questions – Chapter 4

1. What is the keystone of vision? Why is it the keystone?
2. Describe the function of the retina and also where it is located.
3. What is the role of the macula in the eye? What happens during macular degeneration?
4. List the two types of photoreceptors and the function of each one.
5. What is the role of the lens in the eye?
6. Explain the difference between hyperopia, myopia, and astigmatism.
7. What are the diseases of the eye and how are they caused?

CHAPTER 5:

Pressure in the Human Body

Pressure is different in different parts of the body. When breathing in, the pressure in our lungs drops to well below atmospheric. The pressure in our heart when it is beating rises to about 120 mmHg, but when it is returning to the heart the blood pressure is near zero. Our body usually takes care of the very important task of keeping adequate pressures in different parts of the body such as veins, intestines, the bladder, and even our eyes. However, sometimes our body doesn't function properly and problems or diseases can arise when pressure isn't regulated due to injury, genetics, or age.

Units of Pressure

There are many units of pressure that are used in science. Many of these are used in the body. Here are common units:

Pa (Pascal)

Bar

Atm (Atmosphere)

cmH_2O (centimeters of water)

mmHg (millimeters mercury)

lbs/in^2 (pounds per square inch)

Glaucoma

Glaucoma, which was discussed in the last chapter, is a disease caused by increased pressure in the eye, which damages the optic nerve. The front part of the eye is filled with a clear fluid called aqueous humor. This fluid is made behind the iris and exits the eye through channels in the front of the eye in an area called the trabecular meshwork. When this flow of fluid is blocked or slowed, the intraocular pressure will build up and can damage the optic nerve. Glaucoma can occur slowly over time or can happen suddenly due to trauma to the eye. Glaucoma can lead to blindness. Medication can help lower pressure in the eye or surgery can open a new pathway for fluid to drain out of the eye.

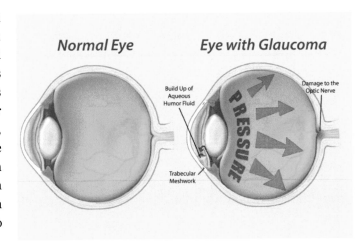

Hiatal Hernia

A hiatal hernia is caused when part of the stomach sticks upward into the chest through a hole in the diaphragm. The hole can be due to injury or weakening of the diaphragm muscle. The condition is very common, especially as patients age, increase in weight, or smoke. Increased pressure in the abdomen caused by heavy lifting, frequent hard coughing and sneezing, pregnancy, straining with constipation, and violent vomiting is also another risk factor for a hernia.

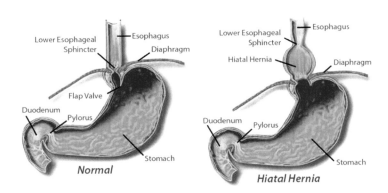

When we breathe, the pressure in the chest decreases to draw air into the lungs. In the case of a hiatal hernia, the decreased pressure in the chest will also draw acid from the stomach into the esophagus. The symptoms of hiatal hernia resemble many other disorders such as dull pains in the chest, shortness of breath, and acid reflux. Surgery is the main way of treating hiatal hernias and restoring the stomach to its correct position in the body. However, medicines such as rantidine, lansoprozale, and omeprazole can also be used to decrease acid levels and tighten the esophagus to prevent the reflux of acid.

Stress Incontinence

When pressure is applied to the abdomen, pressure is likewise applied to the bladder, allowing urine to leak out. Loss of small amounts of urine can also happen when coughing, laughing, sneezing, and exercising. The pressure inside of the bladder increases as it fills. This causes the urethra (and the sphincter that controls urine flow) to move downward, allowing urine to exit. However, when the muscles that support the bladder are weak, the urethra more easily moves down due to increased pressure, allowing urine to exit more easily and frequently. This is why laughing or coughing can cause the leakage of urine. Stress incontinence is a disorder that is mostly seen in women with weakened pelvic floor muscles. The pelvic floor muscles are weakened by pregnancy, childbirth, or menopause as estrogen levels decrease. Treatment includes weight loss and avoiding foods that irritate the bladder such as alcohol, citrus, and spicy foods. Another treatment that increases the effectiveness of the pelvic floor muscles is exercising the muscles through contractions or electrical stimulation. Surgery is very common and is often performed if a woman chooses to have a hysterectomy.

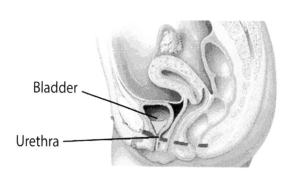

Bladder

Urethra

Varicose Veins

Veins throughout the body have leaflet valves to prevent blood from flowing backwards. However, when these valves are weakened or do not function properly blood can pool and increase pressure in the veins. This condition is called varicose veins and typically occurs in the legs. Varicose veins are often painful, especially while standing or walking. While standing, the superficial veins of the legs are under the most pressure. Fortunately, since varicose veins affect these superficial veins that only supply about 10 percent of the blood back to the heart, surgery can be performed to remove the veins that are not functioning properly. Medications are also available that can shrink the affected blood vessels. Finally, elastic stockings can be worn over the veins to help add counter-pressure and push the pooling blood up out of the legs.

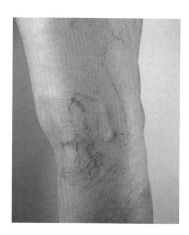

Hydrocephalus

The term hydrocephalus is derived from two Greek words: "hydro," meaning water, and "cephalous," referring to the head. Hydrocephalus is a condition in which excess cerebrospinal fluid (CSF) builds up within the ventricles (which are the fluid-containing cavities) of the brain thus increasing intracranial pressure. Although hydrocephalus is often described as "water on the brain," the "water" is actually CSF. CSF has two crucial functions: acting as a shock absorber for both the brain and spinal cord as well as regulating changes in pressure within the brain. Hydrocephalus can occur at any age but is most common in infants and adults age 60 and older.

Hydrocephalus can be treated in a variety of ways. The problem area may be treated directly by removing the cause of CSF obstruction or indirectly by diverting the fluid to somewhere else (typically to another body cavity) via a shunt. The body cavity in which the CSF is diverted is usually the abdomen. Once inserted, the shunt system usually remains in place for the duration of a patient's life, although additional operations to revise the shunt system are sometimes needed. The shunt system continuously performs its function of diverting the CSF away from the brain, thereby keeping the intracranial pressure within normal limits.

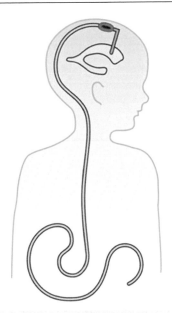

Questions – Chapter 5

1. List some factors that can affect pressure in the body.
2. What is glaucoma and what damage does it cause?
3. What is stress incontinence and how is treated?
4. What is the cause of varicose veins and how are they treated?
5. What is hydrocephalus and how is it treated?

CHAPTER 6:
X-Rays

The Discovery of X-Rays

On November 8, 1895, German physicist Wilhelm Conrad Röntgen (1845-1923) was experimenting with an electric discharge in a vacuum tube when he noticed that as he made sparks in the tube, a fluorescent screen at the other end of the laboratory table glowed slightly. What he determined was that invisible emissions of energy were being produced inside the tube, crossing the room and striking the screen, which produced the faint glimmer. In order to track the progress of the energy emissions, Röntgen placed cards in between the tube and the screen. Nevertheless, the screen continued to glow regardless if the cards were there or not. This meant that the energy emissions were able to pass cleanly through them. He then tried to block the emissions with thin pieces of copper and aluminum. This proved to be just as ineffective as they were as transparent as the cards had been. He then began to place a block of lead right in front of the screen, but dropped it in surprise as he saw the dark skeletal pattern of bones as his hand moved across the face of the screen. Still doubting what he saw, he took out photographic film for a permanent record. Six weeks later, on the Sunday before Christmas 1895, he invited his wife, Bertha, into the laboratory and took a shadowgraph of the bones of her hand with her wedding ring clearly visible.

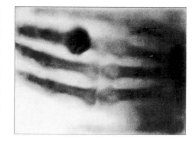

This photograph has become one of the most famous images in photographic and medical history and propelled him within weeks into an international celebrity. The medical implications of his discovery were immediately realized, and the first images of fractured bones were being made by January 1896. Nevertheless, no one yet knew what these mystery energy emissions were.

X-rays are basically the same thing as visible light rays. Both are wavelike forms of **electromagnetic energy** carried by particles called photons. The difference between X-rays and visible light rays is the **energy level** of the individual photons. This is also expressed as the **wavelength** of the rays. Our eyes are sensitive to the particular wavelength of visible light, but not to the shorter wavelength of higher energy X-ray waves or the longer wavelength of the lower energy radio waves. A high frequency X-ray photon carries enough energy that it can break many atomic bonds and even rip molecules apart. The molecular damage caused by X-rays takes time to kill cells. That's why X-ray burns involve little heat and appear long after the exposure.

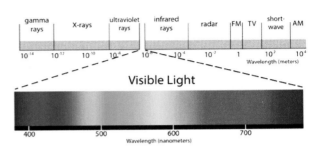

Making X-Rays

Visible light photons and X-ray photons are both produced by the movement of **electrons** in atoms. Electrons occupy different energy levels, or orbitals, around an atom's nucleus. When an electron drops to a lower orbital, it releases energy in the form of a photon. The

Photons are tiny 'packets' of energy and always come in "wavelengths." These wavelengths differ from gamma rays to radio waves. They are the building blocks of light and X-rays.

energy level of the photon depends on how far the electron drops between orbitals, meaning either high or low energy photons can be produced. When a photon collides with another atom, the atom may **absorb** the photon's energy by boosting an electron to a higher level.

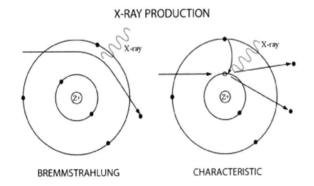

Bremsstrahlung is a German word that means "breaking radiation." This process occurs in an atom when a fast-moving electron emitted from an outside source arcs around a massive nucleus and curves so abruptly that it emits an X-ray photon. How close an electron arcs around the nucleus determines the amount of energy that is emitted in the X-ray photon. The closer an electron comes to the nucleus, the more it accelerates and the more energy it emits. The farther it is, the less it accelerates, and the less energy it emits. That being said, it is more common that an electron arcs further from the nucleus than closer. This means that bremsstrahlung is more likely to produce lower energy X-ray photons than ones of higher energy.

In **characteristic X-ray production,** a fast-moving electron from an outside source collides with an inner orbital electron in a large atom and knocks it completely out of the atom. This collision leaves the atom with a vacant inner orbital that needs to be filled. An electron in an outer orbital fills this vacancy by dropping down to fill it and, in the process, releases an enormous amount of energy. This energy emerges from the atom as an X-ray photon. Because this photon has an energy that's determined by the structure of the atom, it is called a characteristic X-ray and is usually higher in energy than bremsstrahlung X-rays.

An electron volt (eV) is a unit of energy used when discussing the energy of small particles. It is the energy that an electron gains when it travels through a potential (battery or power source) of one volt.

In a typical medical X-ray tube, electrons are emitted by a hot cathode and accelerate through a vacuum toward a positively charged metal anode. The anode is usually made of tungsten or a material called molybdenum and is spun rapidly to keep it from melting. The energy of the electrons as they hit the anode is determined by the voltage difference of the power source. In a medical X-ray machine, the typical voltage difference is about 87,000 V, meaning each electron has about 87,000 electron volts (eV) of energy. When the electrons collide with an atom of tungsten or molybdenum, they emit both bremsstrahlung and characteristic X-rays.

Using X-Rays

X-rays have two important uses in medicine: imaging and radiation therapy. In X-ray imaging, X-rays are sent through a patient's body to a sheet of film or an X-ray detector. While some of the X-rays manage to pass through tissue, most of them are blocked by bone. This means that the patient's bones form a shadow image on the detector behind them. In X-ray radiation therapy, the X-rays are again sent through a patient's body, but now their interaction with diseased tissue is what's important. The X-rays deposit some of their energy in this tissue and kill it. X-ray photons interact with tissue and bone through four major processes: elastic scattering, the photoelectric effect, Compton scattering, and electron-positron pair production.

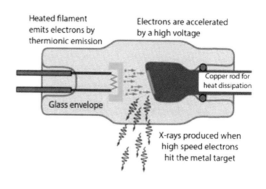

1. **Elastic scattering** is already familiar to us as it is the cause of the blue sky in our atmosphere. Here an atom acts like an antenna for the passing X-ray, letting it pass through without extracting any of its energy. Because this process has almost no effect on the atom, elastic scattering isn't important in radiation therapy. However, it's a nuisance in X-ray imaging because it produces a hazy background because some of the X-rays passing through a patient bounce around like pinballs and arrive at the film from odd angles. To eliminate these bouncing X-ray photons, X-ray machines use filters that block X-rays that don't approach the film from the direction of the X-ray source.

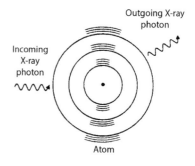

2. **Photoelectric Effect** is when light shines on a metal surface that emits electrons. This is what makes X-ray imaging possible. In this effect, a photon lands on a material, causing an electron of the material to absorb the photon's energy. The electron now has an excess of energy and is tossed completely from the atom. Large atoms such as bone are likely to absorb passing X-rays while small atoms, such as carbon and hydrogen, are likely to let the X-ray photons pass through. That's why bones cast well-defined shadows onto X-ray film while tissue shadows are much less discernable.

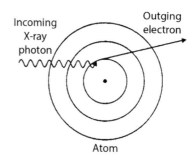

3. **Compton scattering** is where X-rays are used to kill cancer, but they are not the same type of X-rays used for medical imaging. Even though tissue absorbs fewer imaging photons than bone, most imaging photons are absorbed before they can pass through thick tissue. For example, only about 10 percent of imaging photons make it through a patient's leg even when missing the bone. While that percentage is good enough for making an image, it's insufficient for radiation therapy because most imaging X-rays would be absorbed long before

they reached a deep tumor. Instead of killing the tumor, intense exposure to X-rays used for imaging would kill tissue near the patient's skin. In order to attack malignant tissue deep beneath the skin, radiation therapy uses extremely high-energy photons. At photon energies near 1,000,000 eV, the photoelectric effect becomes rare and the photons are much more likely to reach the tumor. Like the photoelectric effect, photons still deposit lethal energy in the tissue and tumor, but they do this through a new effect called Compton scattering. This occurs when an X-ray photon collides with a single electron so that the two particles bounce off one another. The X-ray

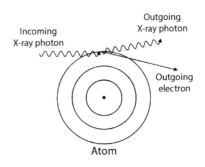

photon ricochets off of the electron while at the same time knocking the electron out of the atom. This process is different from the photoelectric effect because in Compton scattering the photon is bounced, rather than absorbed as it is in the photoelectric effect. The physics behind this effect resembles that of two billiard balls colliding.

Compton scattering is crucial to radiation therapy. When a patient is exposed to 1,000,000 eV photons, most of the photons pass right through them, but a small fraction undergo Compton scattering and leave some of their energy behind. It is this energy that is left behind that kills cancer tissue and can be used to destroy a tumor. By approaching and attacking a tumor from many different angles, the treatment can minimize the injury to healthy tissue around the tumor while giving the tumor itself a fatal dose of radiation.

4. **Electron-positron pair production** is also used to kill cancer. X-rays with slightly more than 1,022,000 eV can cause what is called electron-positron pair production. A positron is the antimatter equivalent of an electron. Almost every particle in nature has an antiparticle with the same mass but with opposite characteristics. A positron has the same mass as an electron, but it is positively charged.

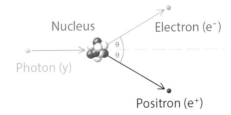

Antimatter doesn't occur naturally on earth, but it can be created in high-energy collisions. When an energetic photon collides with the electric field of an atom, the photon can become an electron and a positron. This event is an example of energy becoming matter. It takes about 511,000 eV of energy to form an electron or a positron, so the photon must have at least 1,022,000 eV to create one of each. Any extra energy goes into kinetic energy in the two particles.

The positron doesn't last long in a patient as it quickly collides with an electron and the two destroy one another as their mass becomes energy. In other words, in electron-positron pair production energy briefly becomes matter and then is turned back into energy. This exotic process is present in high-energy radiation therapy and becomes quite significant at photon energies above about 10,000,000 eV. Not surprisingly, it kills tumors very effectively as well as some surrounding tissue.

Questions – Chapter 6

1. What are X-rays?
2. What are the two types of X-rays created? Describe the production process of each. Which type of X-ray is higher in energy?
3. What are the two medical uses of X-rays?
4. There are four types of X-ray to bone/tissue interaction. What are they? For each type also list the corresponding medical use from the question above.

CHAPTER 7:

Radiation

The word "radiation" sounds ominous and often evokes images of toxic waste fields, cancer, radioactive storage, and nuclear meltdowns. However, many people misunderstand radiation and how it affects living tissue.

There are three primary types of radiation:

- **Alpha** particles are fast moving, high-energy helium atoms. However, due to their large mass, they are stopped by a piece of paper or even just a few inches of air.
- **Beta** particles are fast-moving electrons. Since electrons are less massive than helium atoms, they are able to penetrate through thicker materials. For example, beta particles can penetrate through several feet of air, several millimeters of plastic, or, even more superficially, through very light metals.
- **Gamma** rays, like light or X-rays, are photons except they are much more energetic. X-rays and gamma rays are really the same thing; the difference is how they were produced. Depending on their energy levels, they can be stopped by a thin piece of aluminum foil or penetrate several inches of lead.

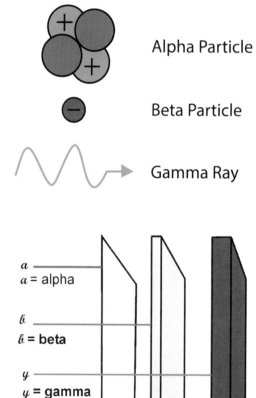

Ionizing and Non-ionizing Radiation

Radiation can be classified as either ionizing or non-ionizing. Non-ionizing radiation is lower energy radiation that comes from the lower part of the electromagnetic spectrum. It is called non-ionizing because it does not have enough energy to completely remove an electron from an atom or molecule. Examples include visible light, infrared light, microwave radiation, and radio waves.

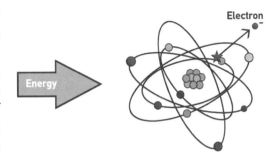

Ionizing radiation has enough energy to break chemical bonds and knock electrons out of atoms, thus changing their net charge. Atoms with missing or extra electrons are called ions, which is why this kind of radiation is called ionizing radiation. It comes from subatomic particles such as alpha and beta particles and the shorter wavelength portion of the electromagnetic spectrum. Examples include ultraviolet, x-rays, and gamma rays.

Atoms prefer to have a net charge of zero, so when they do become charged ions they become unstable. Unstable ions are called free radicals and are much more likely to react with other ions rather than uncharged atoms. Since the body chemistry relies on a finely tuned set of chemical reactions to keep things in balance, these free radicals can interfere and cause damage inside cells. If the damage is too severe, the cells will die. If too many cells are destroyed or damaged at once, such as from a high dose of radiation in a short time period, entire organs can start to fail, eventually leading to death. This is called acute radiation syndrome or radiation poisoning. If the damage isn't too severe or widespread, cells typically have ways of repairing themselves. Unfortunately, sometimes these repairs go wrong, which can still lead to cancer in the long term.

When we measure the amount of radiation that a person is exposed to, the term **Radiation Absorbed Dose** (RADs) is often used.

Radiation Injury

Most damage that is done in living tissues is through ionization. This damage can occur within seconds, but the effects may not be seen for minutes or even decades. The mechanism of injury occurs by either direct or indirect action.

Direct Action (Target Theory) - In this situation, there is a direct hit on the target molecules within the cell. DNA linkage bonds are affected the most and the cell is damaged. This is usually associated with charged particles such as alpha and beta particles.

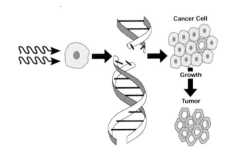

Indirect Action - In this case, radiation leads to splitting of water cells, creating the radicals H_2O^+ and H_2O^-. These two radicals further separate into H^+ and OH^- and interact with membranes, nucleic acids and other enzymes, causing damage to cellular structure and function. This is usually associated with gamma and X-rays.

The real problem is not just the amount of radiation you're exposed to, but rather the amount and kind of radiation that is absorbed over a certain length of time. Alpha particles coming from outside your body are too large and slow to penetrate your skin. Similarly, a few layers of clothing can block beta particles. In contrast, gamma rays can penetrate your body without any trouble, causing more damage. On the other hand, if you were to eat or breathe something that emits alpha or beta particles, the soft tissue inside your body would be affected by that radiation.

A lot of the confusion about how much radiation is 'too much' comes from the fact that scientists use several different units for measuring radiation, depending on exactly what they want to measure about it. More confusing is the fact that some of these units have changed their meanings over the years, and some sources get their conversions between the units mixed up.

Radiation sickness

This is a constellation of health effects that occur within several months of exposure to high amounts of ionizing radiation. The term generally refers to acute medical problems rather than ones that develop after a prolonged period.

The onset and type of symptoms depends on the radiation exposure. As is outlined in the chart below, relatively smaller doses result in gastrointestinal effects such as nausea and vomiting and symptoms related to falling blood counts such as infection and bleeding. Relatively larger doses can result in neurological defects and rapid death. Treatment of acute radiation syndrome is generally performed with blood transfusions and antibiotics. Radiation sickness can be categorized by when the symptoms appear.

- **Prompt effects**, including radiation sickness and radiation burns, may be seen immediately after large doses of radiation are delivered over short periods of time.
- **Delayed effects,** such as cataract formation and cancer, may appear months or years after radiation exposure.

DOSE IN RADS	PROBABLE EFFECT
10 to 50	No obvious effect except possible minor blood changes.
50 to 100	Vomiting and nausea for about one day in 5 percent of exposed persons. No serious reaction. Transient blood problems.
100 to 200	Vomiting and nausea for one day, followed by other symptoms of radiation sickness in 20 to 50 percent of people. No deaths anticipated.
200 to 350	Vomiting and nausea in nearly all people on first day, followed by other symptoms of radiation sickness, loss of appetite, diarrhea and bleeding. About 20 percent will die within six weeks. 75 percent reduction in circulating blood elements.
350 to 550	Vomiting and nausea in most people on the first day, then other radiation sickness symptoms. About 50 percent will die within one month. Survivors will be sick for about six months.
550 to 750	Vomiting and nausea in all people within four hours, followed by severe symptoms of radiation sickness. Up to 100 percent will die.
1000	Vomiting and nausea in all people within one to two hours. All die within days.
5000	Immediate incapacitation. All people will die within one week.

Radiation affects organs differently; the following table is a brief summary of some major organs and the effects of radiation on them.

Brain	Mostly resistant
Skin	Redness and swelling early on, then shriveling of skin followed by skin cancer
Lungs	Breathing difficulty
GI tract	Injury to the lining of the intestines with ulceration
Gonads	Destruction of sperm in testes and destruction of germ cells in the ovaries
Blood and bone marrow	Destruction of red and white blood cells and platelets.

Chapter 7 – Questions

1. What are the three primary types of radiation? Describe their respective penetration energies.
2. What is the difference between ionizing and non-ionizing radiation?
3. With respect to radiation injury, what is the difference between direct and indirect action?
4. What three factors are significant when discussing the severity of radiation injury?
5. Which bodily organ is least affected by radiation?

CHAPTER 8:
The Nervous System

The nervous system is a complex network of nerves and cells that carry messages to and from the brain and spinal cord to various parts of the body. The nervous system includes both the central nervous system (CNS) and peripheral nervous system (PNS). The central nervous system is composed of two kinds of specialized cells called *neurons* and *glial cells*.

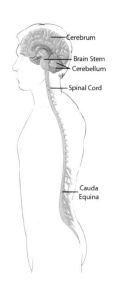

Neuron

The function of a neuron is to receive information from other neurons, process the information, and then send that information to other neurons. This includes all of the motor information by which we are able to move and all of the sensory information through which we are able to see, hear, smell, taste, and touch. This also includes all of the cognitive information through which we are able to reason and think. Processing information requires more than 10,000 different types of neurons, which translates into around 200 billion neurons in the brain alone.

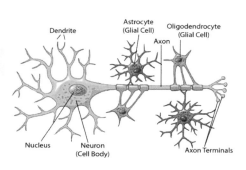

Glial Cells

While we are considering numbers, it is worth noting that there are as many as 50 times more glial cells than neurons in our CNS. Glial cells provide support to the neurons in much the same way that the foundation, framework, and walls of a house provide the structure through which we run various electrical outlets, pipes, and telephone lines. Not only do glial cells provide the structural framework that allow networks of neurons to remain connected, they also attend to the brain's various housekeeping functions such as removing debris after neuronal death.

Structure of Neurons

While there are as many as 10,000 specific types of neurons, they are generally divided into three general types:

1. *Motor neurons*–transmit information about muscle motion
2. *Sensory neurons*– transmit sensory information
3. *Interneurons*–transmit information between different types of neurons

A typical neuron has four distinct parts. The first part is the cell body and is the control center of the neuron.

The second is called the axon, and the third is called the dendrite. These are structures that extend away from the cell body, acting as conduits through which signals flow to or away from the cell body. Incoming signals are received through the dendrites. The outgoing signal to other neurons flows along the axon. A neuron may have many thousands of dendrites, but it will have only one axon.

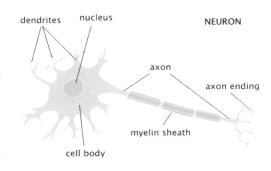

The fourth distinct part of a neuron lies at the end of the axon. These are the axon terminals and are the structures that contain neurotransmitters. Neurotransmitters are the chemicals that are released into the synapses that communicate with the next neuron. A low level of neurotransmitters is the cause of depression. Drugs such as Prozac, Lexapro, and Celexa aim at helping to raise the level of neurotransmitters in order to cure depression.

Another important structure of the neuron is a covering called the myelin sheath. This is a segmented covering around axons and dendrites of peripheral neurons. This casing is continuous along axons except at regular gaps called the nodes of Ranvier. The myelin sheath aids in moving nerve impulses much more rapidly than would otherwise be possible.

Action Potential

Action potential is the process by which nerve impulses travel along the nervous system and thus through the body. Neurons send messages electrochemically, meaning that chemicals within the body cause an electrical signal. Chemicals in the body that are electrically charged are called ions. The important ions in the nervous system

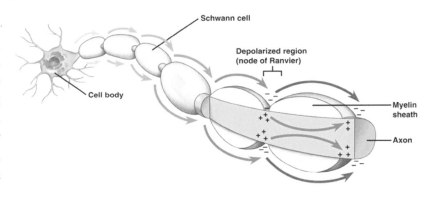

are sodium and potassium. By passing these ions through the semi-permeable membrane of the node of Ranvier, an electrical signal can be conducted.

Nerve impulses occur like a domino effect. Each neuron receives an impulse and must pass it on to the next neuron. Through a chain of chemical events, dendrites receive an impulse, which then travels through the axon and is transmitted to the next neuron. The entire nerve impulse passes through a neuron in about seven milliseconds — faster than a lightning strike.

When a neuron is not stimulated, its membrane is polarized, which means that the electrical charge on the outside of the membrane is positive while the electrical charge on the inside of the membrane is negative. The outside of the cell has an excess of sodium ions (Na+), while the inside of the cell contains excess potassium ions (K+).

When the neuron is inactive or polarized, it's said to be at its resting potential. It remains this way until a stimulus arrives. When the stimulus occurs, sodium ions move inside the membrane and potassium moves out. This rush of ions moving in and out of the axon stimulates the next section of the neuron to do the same thing and consequently creates a motion down the axon called the action potential.

The speed of a nerve impulse varies with the type the nervous system is sending. Nerve impulses such as pain travel slowly at 0.6 m/s. Touch signals travel at speeds of 76 m/s. Thought signals are traveling at 30 meters per second. Signals that help to determine spatial perception travel at speeds up to 120 m/s. But even the fastest nerve impulses are three million times slower than the speed of electricity through a wire.

Electrical Conduction in the Heart

An action potential is generated in the heart similar to the rest of the body. It starts high up in the upper right atrium at a bundle of cells called the sinoatrial (SA) node. This is the natural pacemaker of the heart. You may have heard of someone having a pacemaker implanted in his or her body when the SA node has ceased to function properly. The SA node releases electrical signals at a rate that is determined by the needs of the body (usually that is between 60 – 100 times each minute). Each signal passes through the heart cells, creating a wave of contraction that spreads rapidly through both of the atrium. When a person is exercising, the SA node is stimulated to beat faster, as high as 180 – 190 times per minute.

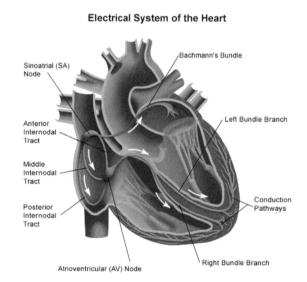

Electrical System of the Heart

The electrical stimulus from the SA node eventually reaches another bundle of special cells in the lower part of the right atrium called the atrioventricular (AV) node. Once the atria are empty of blood, the valves between the atria and ventricles close. At this point, the electrical stimulus passes out of the AV node into a special set of nerves called the bundle of His, and then into another set of nerves called the Purkinje fibers. Imagine the bundle of His as a highway, with the Purkinje fibers being roads that spread widely across the ventricles. In this way all the cells in in the ventricles receive an electrical stimulus, causing them to contract.

Most people have seen an electrical reading of the heart called an EKG. There are usually five waves on an EKG labeled P, Q, R, S and T. The P wave shows the electrical impulse starting at the SA node and proceeding through the atria, causing the atria to contract. The QRS waves are indicative of the impulse going through the ventricles starting at the AV node, causing the ventricles to contract. The T wave displays repolarization, that is, the resetting of the conducting system for the next impulse.

Pain

Pain is one of the products of having an advanced nervous system. While pain protects us from harm, it outlasts its usefulness. For example, we can put our hand on a hot stove and our nervous system can warn us of danger through the pain, but the pain can still linger long after we remove our hand.

Because of this, our bodies have developed two natural defenses against pain. First, a chemical called endorphins can be released from the brain. These endorphins act like pain medication, reducing sharp and severe pain for short periods of time by covering up pain with a warm, insensible feeling. This is what allows a football player to continue towards the end zone to score a touchdown, seemingly oblivious to the fact he broke his arm at the beginning of the play.

The second way our bodies deal with pain is called "gating." Our brain can be thought of as an airport, with planes always arriving and departing. These planes are the signals sent by nerves that they are detecting pain or some sort of feeling or touch. However, the brain can only handle one sensation landing at a time, much like some small airports with only one runway. This means that the dominant sensation will be the only one registered in our brains and all others will be blocked out and seemingly non-existent for a time. Hence the many remedies that we try when we are experiencing pain, such as rubbing our temples when we have a headache, or massaging and shaking the finger or hand that we just accidentally smashed with a heavy object. This is the same type of strategy that ice packs and heating pads are used for. When we create a sensation that overpowers pain, we only feel the sensation that was created and not the pain.

Lidocaine is a drug that physicians and dentists use to numb an area they are about to work on. It works by blocking the channels at the nodes of Ranvier that allow the influx of sodium preventing the action potential from working. No action potential means that there is no nerve impulse. If you inject Lidocaine next to a motor neuron, it will create a temporary paralysis.

Diseases of the Nervous System

Multiple Sclerosis (MS) is an autoimmune disease that affects the brain and central nervous system. Generally, MS is caused by damage to the myelin sheath. When the sheath is damaged, nerve signals slow down and even stop. Some of the symptoms of MS include loss of balance, muscle spasms, numbness, problems walking, tremors, double vision, and even vision loss. There are also symptoms associated with the bowels, the bladder, speech, and swallowing.

While a specific cause has not been identified, MS has been linked to a combination of genetic, environmental, and infectious factors. There is no cure for MS, but some treatments have proven somewhat effective for helping affected individuals achieve a better quality of life than otherwise possible. Medications can be used to slow the progression of the disease, decrease the severity of attacks, and control the symptoms.

Lou Gehrig's disease is another illness that can affect the way electrical signals are produced and relayed through the body. Its real name is Amyotrophic Lateral Sclerosis (ALS). The disorder is marked by rapid and progressive muscle weakness and atrophy that leads to difficulty speaking, swallowing and breathing as the neurons that control these movements and muscles are destroyed. There is also no known cause for ALS with patients who have no previous family history of ALS. However, there is some evidence that head trauma from contact sports or chemical or electromagnetic field exposure can cause ALS. Recently there have been studies that have shown genetics may play a more important role in the cause of the disease. There is no cure for ALS.

Questions – Chapter 8

1. What are the two specialized cells that compose the central nervous system?
2. List the three general types of neurons and their functions.
3. What are the four distinct parts of a neuron and what is the function of each part?
4. What is the purpose of the myelin sheath?
5. What is action potential and how does it work in the body?
6. Explain the action potential of the heart and how this causes it to beat.
7. List the diseases of the nervous system and some of the causes and symptoms of each.
8. What are the two ways the body 'defends' itself against pain?

CHAPTER 9:
Neuroscience

Structure of the Brain

The human brain is the most complex organ in the body and controls our every thought and action. It is a pinkish-beige in color and weighs about 3 pounds (as much as a half gallon of milk). It is very soft to the touch. The brain is divided into left and right hemispheres, which are almost identical in structure. Each side has four lobes - the frontal lobe, temporal lobe, parietal lobe, and occipital lobe. Each lobe controls different functions of the body. The brain is connected to the spinal cord via the brain stem, which also regulates metabolic activity in the body. The cerebellum (Latin for "little brain") is located where the brain connects to the brain stem and is primarily responsible for motor skills. The brain is covered in wrinkles or folds to increase its surface area to accommodate the high function processing needs of humans. If we were to stretch out the brain to undo all of the folds, it would be about the size of a pillowcase.

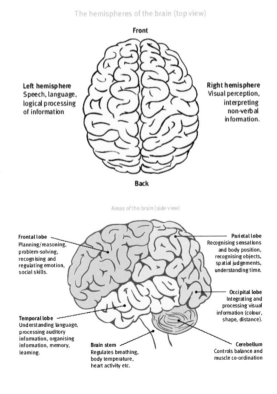

The hemispheres of the brain (top view)

Front

Left hemisphere
Speech, language, logical processing of information

Right hemisphere
Visual perception, interpreting non-verbal information.

Back

Areas of the brain (side view)

Frontal lobe
Planning/reasoning, problem-solving, recognising and regulating emotion, social skills.

Parietal lobe
Recognising sensations and body position, recognising objects, spatial judgements, understanding time.

Occipital lobe
Integrating and processing visual information (colour, shape, distance).

Temporal lobe
Understanding language, processing auditory information, organising information, memory, learning.

Brain stem
Regulates breathing, body temperature, heart activity etc.

Cerebellum
Controls balance and muscle co-ordination

Why Do We Have a Brain?

We need brains not so much to think, but rather, in order to move. Think about this for a minute. Today, humans have been able to create computers that can beat the smartest chess player in the world, in fact, it was done years ago with very simple computers. However the most sophisticated and advanced computers cannot make motion. That is, the best of all computers can barely grab a glass of water and lift it, without breaking it. That's it, nothing else!

Another example of the brains incredible ability to make us move is shown in a small ocean animal called a sea squirt. This little thing is born with a brain and a nervous system. Using its brain, it moves through the ocean until it finds a piece of coral to live on. Once it permanently plants itself, it digests its own brain and nervous system, and then lives on food that flows through the ocean current. It no longer moves, so it no longer needs its brain for movement, so it eats it.

Movement and becoming more athletic has driven the need for a bigger more complicated brain. In 2004, biologists Daniel E. Lieberman of Harvard and Dennis M. Bramble and David Carrier of the University of Utah showed that our ancestors survived by becoming endurance athletes, able to bring down swifter prey through sheer doggedness, jogging and plodding along behind them until the animals dropped from exhaustion.

Endurance produced meals, which provided energy for mating, which meant that adept early joggers passed along their genes. In this way, natural selection drove early humans to develop longer legs, shorter toes, new tendons, less hair and complicated inner-ear mechanisms to maintain balance and stability during upright walking. Being in motion made humans smarter, and being smarter allowed them to move more efficiently. Movement shaped the human body and that shaped the human brain.

Because of this, humans became smarter with the brains increasing rapidly in size. Today, humans have a brain that is about three times the size that would be expected. So physical activity has played a critical role in making our brains larger and physical activity helped to make humans smarter. Out of all of this came the ability to understand higher math, read, explore and even invent iPads.

The broad point of this is that physical activity helped to mold the structure of our brains. So movement and physical activity remain essential to brain health today. And there is scientific support for that idea. Recent studies have shown that regular exercise, even walking, leads to more robust mental abilities, from childhood into old age.

The Working Brain

Everything we do relies on neurons communicating with one another. Electrical impulses and chemical signals carrying messages across different parts of the brain and between the brain and the rest of the nervous system. When a neuron is activated a small difference in electrical charge occurs. This unbalanced charge is called an action potential and is caused by the concentration of ions (atoms or molecules with unbalanced charges) across the cell membrane. The action potential travels very quickly along the axon, like when a line of dominoes falls.

When the action potential reaches the end of an axon, most neurons release a chemical message (a neurotransmitter) which crosses the synapse and binds to receptors on the receiving neuron's dendrites and starts the process over again. At the end of the line, a neurotransmitter may stimulate a different kind of cell (like a gland cell), or may trigger a new chain of messages.

Neurotransmitters send chemical messages between neurons. Mental illnesses, such as depression, can occur when this process does not work correctly. Communication between neurons can also be electrical, such as in areas of the brain that control movement. When electrical signals are abnormal, they can cause tremors or symptoms found in Parkinson's disease.

Serotonin—helps control many functions, such as mood, appetite, and sleep. Research shows that people with depression often have lower than normal levels of serotonin. The types of medications most commonly prescribed to treat depression act by blocking the recycling, or reuptake, of serotonin by the sending neuron. As a result, more serotonin stays in the synapse for the receiving neuron to bind onto, leading to more normal mood functioning.

Dopamine—mainly involved in controlling movement and aiding the flow of information to the front of the brain, which is linked to thought and emotion. It is also linked to reward systems in the brain. Problems in producing dopamine can result in Parkinson's disease, a disorder that affects a person's ability to move as they want to, resulting in stiffness, tremors or shaking, and other symptoms. Some studies suggest that having too little dopamine or problems using dopamine in the thinking and feeling regions of the brain may play a role in disorders like schizophrenia or attention deficit hyperactivity disorder (ADHD)

Glutamate—the most common neurotransmitter, glutamate has many roles throughout the brain and nervous system. Glutamate is an excitatory transmitter: when it is released it increases the chance that the neuron will fire. This enhances the electrical flow among brain cells required for normal function and plays an important role during early brain development. It may also assist in learning and memory. Problems in making or using glutamate have been linked to many mental disorders, including autism, obsessive compulsive disorder (OCD), schizophrenia, and depression.

Meet Sarah

Sarah is a college student who seemed to have it all. Then, after a serious setback at home, she lost interest in her studying. She had problems getting to sleep and generally felt tired, listless, and had no appetite most of the time. Weeks later, Sarah realized she was having trouble coping with the stresses in her life. She began to think of suicide because she felt like things weren't going to get better and that there was nothing she could do about it.

Worried at the changes she saw, Sarah's mother took her to the doctor, who ran some tests. After deciding her symptoms were not caused by a stroke, brain tumor, or similar conditions, Sarah's doctor referred her to a psychologist.

The psychologist asked Sarah about symptoms and family medical history. It's important to remember that everyone gets "the blues" from time to time. In contrast, major depression is a serious disorder that lasts for weeks. Sarah told the doctor that she had experienced long periods of deep sadness throughout her teenage years, but had never seen a doctor about it. She has faced a few bouts since then, but they have never been as bad as her current mood.

The psychologist diagnosed Sarah with major depression and gave her a prescription for a type of antidepressant medication called a selective serotonin reuptake inhibitor (SSRI). SSRIs are the most common type of medication used to treat depression. SSRIs boost the amount of serotonin in the brain and help reduce symptoms of depression. Sarah also has several follow-up visits scheduled with the psychologist to check how she's responding to the treatment. She also begins regular talk therapy sessions with her psychologist. In these sessions, she learns how to change the way she thinks about and reacts to things that may trigger her depression. Several months later, Sarah feels much better. She continues taking SSRIs and has joined an online support group. Sharing her experiences with others also dealing with depression helps Sarah to better cope with her feelings.

Memory

Researches have been studying memory for as long as, well, as long as people can remember. The most common image of memory is a type of filing cabinet filled with memory folders where data is pulled out, or as a super computer with infinite random access storage. But it turns out that this is not correct. A better image might be a complex spider web with data stored all over the entire brain. The simple act of riding a bike will require that the brain retrieve information that it has stored in possibly millions of places.

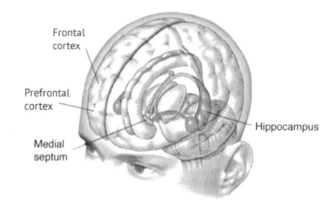

Memory begins with perception. Experts believe that the hippocampus, along with another part of the brain called the frontal cortex, is responsible for analyzing these various sensory inputs and deciding if they're worth remembering. If they are, they may become part of your long-term memory.

Memories are encoded and stored using the language of electricity and chemicals through trillions of points called a synapse. All the action in your brain occurs at these synapses, where electrical pulses carrying messages leap across gaps between cells.

To properly encode a memory, you must first be paying attention. Since you cannot pay attention to everything all the time, most of what you encounter every day is simply filtered out, and only a few stimuli pass into your conscious awareness. If you remembered every single thing that you noticed, your memory would be full before you even left the house in the morning. What scientists aren't sure about is whether stimuli are screened out during the sensory input stage or only after the brain processes its significance. What we do know is that how you pay attention to information may be the most important factor in how much of it you actually remember.

After that first flicker, the sensation is stored in short-term memory. Short-term memory has a fairly limited capacity; it can hold about seven items for no more than 20 or 30 seconds at a time. You may be able to increase this capacity somewhat by using various memory strategies. Important information is gradually transferred from short-term memory into long-term memory. The more the information is repeated or used, the more likely it is to eventually end up in long-term memory, or to be retained. That's why studying helps people to perform better on tests. Unlike short-term memory, long-term memory can store unlimited amounts of information indefinitely.

People tend to more easily store material on subjects that they already know something about, since the information has more meaning to them and can be mentally connected to related information that is already stored in their long-term memory. That's why someone who has an average memory may be able to remember a greater depth of information about one particular subject.

Have you and a friend every argued over recalling the same event differently? This happens a lot because memories change. Each time you recall something, it will be different than the last time you recalled it. Our brains are constantly betraying us, transforming our memories every time we think about them. That is because every memory we have is colored by the times we've recollected it before. It's a lot like Wikipedia with an autocorrect function, you can change it, and so can someone else.

Recalling a memory more often makes that memory less accurate, and that every time you take a memory off the shelf in your brain, you put it back just a tiny bit different. That's because instead of remembering the actual memory, you're recalling the memory of the last time you remembered it and any mistakes that might have been introduced there. A memory is not simply an image produced by time traveling back to the original event—it is an image that is somewhat distorted because of the prior times you remembered it. Memory of an event grows less precise even to the point of being totally false. This fact is responsible for putting a lot of innocent people in jail. Today most people outsource their memory to smart phones and electronics that has the great affect of freeing up space for other tasks.

The Strange Case of Henry Molaison

Henry Molaison was a 27-year-old man who suffered from severe epileptic seizures. The year was 1953 and brain surgery was still in its infancy. The treatment decided upon, however, was to remove large parts of Molaison's brain where the seizures occurred. Most of the area removed was the hippocampus the brain's memory center, where short-term memory is converted into long-term memory. In the first hours after waking from surgery he appeared normal. He was cordial to the hospital staff and seemed to have no major cognitive deficits as a result of the surgery. But upon meeting someone new he could only converse normally as long as the person never left the room. If they left the room for just a few minutes it was as if Molaison had never met them. They would come back into the room and have to reintroduce themselves. Upon closer analysis the doctors realized that he could still recall facts that he'd known prior to the surgery but he could no longer form new memories. He could, at most, hold information for only several minutes before it was lost to him forever. He was now suffering from a very sorrowful plight, he would never again form a new memory. Molaison could keep information for several minutes in short-term memory. His long-term memory was intact too, as he could remember things he'd learned prior to the surgery. The fact that he still retained both short - and long-term memories but could form no new long-term memories proved that the hippocampus was crucial to converting short-term memory into long-term memory. Molaison was never able to live independently after the surgery. He lived with his parents, tending to simple chores like going to the grocery store and spending hours with his crossword puzzles. Having been 27 at the time of the surgery, he never got used to the graying person that greeted him in the mirror every morning decades later and looked in horror at himself, wondering what was happening. He died at age 82.

The Teenage Brain

It had always been assumed that the vast majority of brain development took place in the first few years of life. Recently neuroscientists have learned that this is not the case. Using structural MRI to look at size and functional MRI (called fMRI) to look at brain activity, we now have a detailed picture of how the brain actually develops throughout

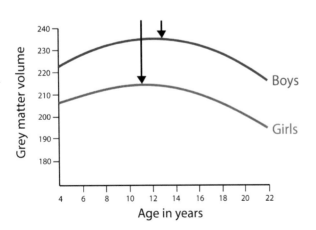

adolescence and even into the 20's. Adolescence is defined as the period of life that starts with the biological, hormonal, physical changes of puberty and ends at the age at which an individual attains a stable, independent role in society. One part of the brain that changes the most dramatically during adolescence is called the prefrontal cortex (located in front of the frontal cortex, as seen in the *Memory* section). This is a very interesting brain area. It's proportionally much bigger in humans than in any other species, and it's involved in a whole range of high level cognitive functions, such as decision-making, planning what you're going to do tomorrow or next week or next year, inhibiting inappropriate behavior, such as stopping yourself saying something really rude or doing something really stupid. It is also involved in social interaction, understanding other people, and self-awareness.

MRI studies looking at the development of this region have shown that it really undergoes dramatic development during the period of adolescence. The size of this region increases during childhood and peaks in early adolescence. The peak happens a couple of years later in boys relative to girls since boys start puberty several years later. During adolescence, there's a significant decline in volume in the prefrontal cortex. Now that might sound bad, but actually this is a really important developmental process. Gray matter contains cell bodies and also connections between the cells, called synapses. This decline in volume during adolescence is thought to correspond to synaptic pruning, that is, the elimination of unwanted synapses. This is a really important process. It's partly dependent on the environment that the human is in. The synapses that are being used are strengthened, and synapses that aren't being used are pruned away. You can think of it a bit like pruning a rosebush. You prune away the weaker branches so that the remaining, important branches can grow stronger. This process very effectively fine-tunes brain tissue during the period of adolescence.

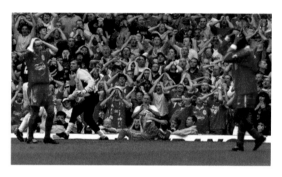

The prefrontal cortex is also the area of the brain that we use to understand other people and to interact with other people. The photograph of the soccer game illustrates two aspects of how our social brains work. This is a soccer game in which the great soccer player, Michael Owen, has just missed a goal. He is lying on the ground. The first aspect of the social brain that this picture illustrates is how automatic and instinctive social emotional responses are. Within a split second of Michael Owen missing this goal, everyone is doing the same thing with their arms and the same thing with their face. The second aspect of the social brain that this picture nicely illustrates is just how good we are at reading other people's behavior, their actions, their gestures, their facial expressions, in terms of their underlying emotions and mental states. So you don't have to ask any of these people what they are feeling. You already have a pretty good idea.

Studies show that a teenager's ability to take into account someone else's ideas in order to guide their own behavior is still developing well into late adolescence. In addition, we know that adolescents have a tendency to take risks. They take more risks than children or adults, and they are particularly prone to taking risks when they're with their friends. There's an important drive to become independent from one's parents and to impress one's friends in adolescence. We can try to understand this in terms of the development of a part of their brain called the limbic system. It is located deep inside the brain, and it's involved in things like emotion processing and reward processing. It gives us the kick out of taking risks. The limbic system has been found to be hypersensitive to the rewarding feeling of risk-taking in adolescents compared with adults, and at the very same time, the prefrontal cortex, which stops us taking excessive risks, is still very much in development in adolescents. This helps us to explain why teens take risks, whereas adults do not.

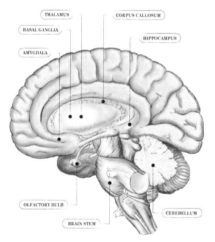

THE LIMBIC SYSTEM

Research has shown that the adolescent brain undergoes really quite profound development, and this has implications for education, for rehabilitation, and teaching. The environment shapes the developing adolescent brain. This is a fantastic opportunity for learning and creativity. So what's sometimes seen as the problem with adolescents — heightened risk-taking, poor impulse control, self-consciousness — shouldn't be stigmatized. It actually reflects changes in the brain that provide amazing opportunities to educate and change.

Optical Illusions

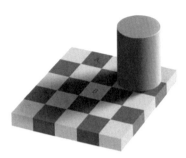

The world presents us with a constant stream of visual information that we must perceive and process. Our eyes are the tools that help us in gathering this visual information, but in the end our brain is actually what sees and makes sense of all this information. Optical illusions demonstrate how, even when visual information enters through the eye properly, the brain can process it incorrectly and cause us to experience an object or environment differently than how it is actually displayed.

An optical illusion is a mismatch between the immediate visual impression and the actual properties of the object. Optical illusions occur when visually perceived images differ from what is actually present in objective reality. As was already said, this happens when the eye gathers information and sends it to the brain, which processes the information in a way that does not correlate to the actual state of a given object. There are three types of visual illusions: literal optical illusions, physiological illusions, and cognitive illusions.

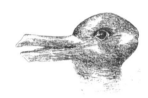

- Literal optical illusions are images created in our brain that are different from the objects they represent.
- Physiological illusions are the result of effects on the eyes and brain of excessive stimulation of a specific type such as brightness, color, size, position, tilt, movement, etc.
- Cognitive illusions are the result of unconscious inferences. i.e., they occur because the brain unconsciously uses other objects to compare and perceive size, shape, and color.

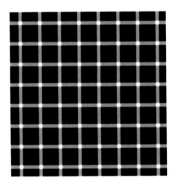

Optical illusions occur due to properties of the visual areas of the brain as they receive and process information. In other words, your perception of an illusion has more to do with how your brain works and less to do with the optics of your eye. For years now, scientists and researchers have known that there is a delay of one-tenth of a second between the time that light hits our eye and the time the light impulse arrives at our brain and is processed into an image. While one-tenth of a second is not a large delay, it is enough that the brain tries to predict what the eyes are going to see.

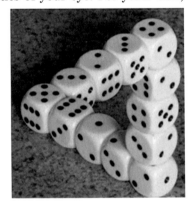

As we age and have new experiences, our brain stores information of how things should feel, smell, and hear. It also stores visual information about how things are supposed to appear. This means that as we see things, our brain subconsciously fills in parts of our field of vision. In other words, our brains are constantly trying to see the future and create an image based on learned expectations.

Diseases of Brain and Thought

Alzheimer's disease – Alzheimer's disease is a progressive neurologic disease of the brain leading to the irreversible loss of neurons and the loss of intellectual abilities, including memory and reasoning, which become severe enough to impede social or occupational functioning. During the course of the disease *plaque* sand *tangles* develop within the structure of the brain. This causes brain cells to die. Patients with Alzheimer's also have a deficiency in the levels of some vital brain chemicals that are involved with the transmission of messages in the brain called neurotransmitters.

Alzheimer's disease is the most common form of **dementia**. The disease gets worse with time. There is no current cure for Alzheimer's, although there are ways of slowing down its advance and helping patients with some of the symptoms. Alzheimer's is also a terminal disease - it is incurable and causes death.

There are estimated to be between 2.5 million and 4.5 million Americans who have Alzheimer's. **One third of all seniors in America die with Alzheimer's or some other dementia** according to the Alzheimer's Association. Deaths from Alzheimer's have risen by 68% from 2000 to 2010.

People who lead active lifestyles and exercise regularly are more likely to slow down the progression of Alzheimer's disease while active people who are Alzheimer's free have a lower risk of developing the disease or any kind of dementia.

Schizophrenia - Schizophrenia is a mental condition that distorts one's perception of reality and causes hallucinations, desire for seclusion, and often, violence. The Greek word Schizophrenia directly translates to "split mind" which is ironic, because those with the mental disorder barely have one personality, let alone multiple, as the term suggests. This mental disorder is caused by an imbalance of dopamine in the brain. Drugs are available that correct the dopamine levels, but treatment is not entirely effective because some patients refuse to cooperate, are unaffected by the drugs, or experience drastic side affects. Studies have shown that Schizophrenia is sometimes associated with minor differences in brain structure, including reduced volume of the frontal and temporal lobes. It is unknown, however, if these structural differences are present before the onset of the disorder, or if they develop over time. Those with Schizophrenia are likely to have other mental disorders, such as depression or anxiety, and often have long-term social handicaps. Many don't have the capacity to hold a job and instead seek isolation on the streets.

Parkinson's disease - Parkinson's disease affects the electrical impulses of the nervous system and is somewhat similar to MS and ALS. Parkinson's disease is characterized by a slowing of voluntary movements, muscular rigidity, and tremors while the body is at rest. These symptoms are caused by a reduction of neurons responsible for making dopamine in the brain. This in turn can affect how other neurons fire and react to different stimuli, especially those nerves and neurons that control the muscles and limbs of your body.

Artificial Intelligence

Artificial intelligence (often abbreviated as AI) is the broad field of computer science that attempts to make computers deal with complex situations in the way a human would behave.

The Turing Test

AI is as old as computer science itself. In fact, the oldest, most famous and possibly loftiest challenge of the field is called the Turing Test named after Alan Turing, the father of modern computing. In 1950, he considered this question: can machines think? Because humans and machines "think" very differently, he suggested a simple experiment that could serve as a proxy for the answer to that question and though called it the *imitation game*, it's come to be known as the *Turing Test*.

It goes like this: an average person sits down at a computer and has an instant message conversation with two other people. The catch is that one of them is not a human, but rather a computer designed to give human-like answers. If this person cannot determine which conversation is with a real person, then the computer giving the responses has passed the Turing Test.

Computer Chess

So how does artificial intelligence work? It's an expansive field of computer science and there's no single answer to that question, but a very common form of artificial intelligence can be demonstrated with a discussion of a simple game: computer chess. For a very long time this drove a lot of innovation in artificial intelligence among both hobbyists and even large and innovative companies like IBM. Starting in the 1970s, computer chess conventions were regularly held in major cities where enthusiasts would pit computer against computer in very serious AI chess matches. The winners would ultimately be determined not only the speed of the computer but by the quality of AI that chose the chess moves.

Check Mate: Machine vs. Human

While computers were becoming increasingly sophisticated in the way they played against other computers, it took a very long time for a computer to match the skills of the world's chess grandmasters. That finally ended in 1997 when Deep Blue, a super computer created by IBM, was finally able to beat Garry Kasparov (then a world champion and still considered by some to be the greatest chess player of all time). Interestingly, Deep Blue may have beat Garry Kasparov only because of a software bug. At a critical point in the first game of the series, Deep Blue ran into an unanticipated situation and fell back to making a random move. This move surprised Kasparov who interpreted it as a new level of advancement in artificial intelligence. He managed to win that first game, but it seemed to shake his confidence. In the end, Kasparov and Deep Blue tied one game, Kasparov won two, and Deep Blue won three, marking the first time that a computer had beaten the a grandmaster in an official series.

There are many remarkable things to consider in that story, but the most remarkable question might be this: how did Kasparov and other chess masters beat machines for so long? Computers are able to evaluate millions of possibilities each second whereas human brains can only consciously evaluate one or two things in that much time.

Human Computing

It's tempting to think of the operation of our brains as being a lot like that of a computer. Computers, after all, appear to "think" when they are performing long tasks. But how do our brains really compare to the RAM and CPUs that power the computers we use every day? In reality they are very different. The CPUs in modern computers process very simple commands that we call instructions. Examples are adding two numbers together or fetching a number from memory. When thousands or millions of these instructions are executed in sequence, they become a program or an application and can accomplish incredibly complex and interesting tasks. When you buy a computer with a CPU that runs at 3.4 Ghz, that means that the CPU can execute about 3.4 billion instructions per second. That's a lot of math! By comparison, most neurons in the human brain can only fire five or six times per second. That means that a computer's CPU is literally millions of times faster than a neuron.

Parallel Processing

So how did the brain of a chess player outperform the world's faster computers for so many years? What the brain lacks in speed, it makes up in numbers. There are an estimated 100 billion neurons in the human brain. Each of those millions of neurons can work together, many functioning at the same time, to create a sophisticated information processing mesh that is unlike any modern computer in its ability to identify, store and access information. This is a huge advantage. Computers process information linearly. In our chess example, that means that each move and all of its implications must be considered individually. A computer can literally only think about one thing at a time. This can be a little like trying to play a symphony one note at a time.

The human brain, on the other hand, can process complete and meaningful ideas all at once as the information spreads across a dense mesh of billions of neurons. As the brain encounters new information, it forms connections between neurons. If it encounters the same (or similar) stimuli again, those connections get reinforced. Eventually, the neurons become attuned to certain patterns and those patterns become the basis for knowledge, reasoning and learning. This gives the human brain nearly instant access to incredibly complex and different ideas and patterns. A computer plays a symphony one note at a time, the brain can access the entire full orchestra.

Pattern Matching

How does an athlete know how to catch a ball? A computer might perform this task through complex mathematical calculations. Humans do something much differently. We look for patterns. And our brains are adept at finding them. When a football is hurling through the air at an all-star running back, the player's brain isn't doing the physics calculations that a computer might do. Instead, it's matching patterns. It has seen a ball in a air like that before and it knows where it's going to be next and makes the hands go to that spot.

The Future of Artificial Intelligence

The future of AI is and always has been a controversial topic. The closer machines come to "thinking" the less comfortable we seem to feel about the role they play in our lives. On the other hand, innovations in artificial intelligence over the last few decades have created indispensable technology that has touched our lives nearly every day, including everything from spam filters and video games to medical research and mapping technology. In the future, machines may use AI to drive our cars and prepare our meals.

Questions – Chapter 9

1. Name the four lobes of the brain and briefly describe the function of each.
2. What is the main reason why we have brains?
3. Why don't we remember everything we see?
4. Why is it that two people can have different recollections of the same event?
5. In your own words, describe what optical illusions are and how/why we see them.
6. Which diseases of the brain are caused by dopamine imbalances?

CHAPTER 10:

Physics of Bones and Trauma

Bones

Bones are amazing in that they can last for centuries and in some cases for millions of years. Since they are strong, humans have used them for tools, weapons, and even art. In order for our bodies to function, bones have to be incredibly versatile. Nature has solved this problem extremely well by varying the shapes and the types of bones in our bodies. If you sorted all of the approximately 200 bones of the body into various piles according to their shapes, you might come up with four piles. First would be a small pile of flat, plate-like bones such as the shoulder blade (scapula) and some of the bones of the skull. The second pile would consist of long, hollow bones such as those found in the arms, legs, and fingers. A third pile would have more or less cylindrical bones from the spine (vertebrae), and a fourth pile would have irregular bones such as those from the wrist and ankle.

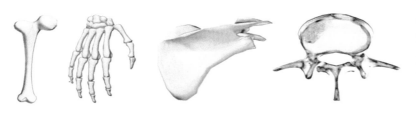

Bones serve very important purposes in our bodies:

1. **Support**: Simply put, bones support the body. They are the foundation to which many things in our bodies anchor. For example, tendons and ligaments attach directly to bone and help to hold us together. In certain diseases some of this support structure deteriorates.

2. **Movement**: Joints permit the movement of our bones and are very important for many of the motions of the body. We can manage with some loss of joint movement, but the destruction of joints by arthritis can seriously limit mobility.

3. **Protection of organs**: Protection of vital organs is a very important function of some bones. The skull protects the brain and several of the most important sensory organs like the eyes and ears. The ribs form a protective cage for the heart, lungs, and liver. In addition to its support role, the spinal column serves as a flexible shield for the spinal cord.

4. **Storage of chemicals**: Bones act as a bank for storing chemicals for future use by the body that can be withdrawn as needed. For example, a minimum level of calcium is needed in the blood, so if the level falls too low, a calcium sensor causes the parathyroid glands to release more parathyroid hormone into the blood, which in turn causes the bones to release needed calcium.

5. **Function**: The teeth are specialized bones that cut, tear, and grind the food that we eat. The smallest bones in the body are found in the middle ear and contribute to the ability to hear. These three small bones act as levers that convert sound vibrations in the air to sound vibrations in the fluid in the cochlea. The ribs serve as a bellows, opening and closing the lungs to move air in and out of our bodies, meaning that bones help us to breathe.

Bone is a living tissue that contains nerves and requires a blood supply. If this blood supply is diminished or stopped, bone can die. For example, a serious hip problem is caused by a condition called avascular necrosis in which the bone cells in the hip die due to a lack of blood. Cells called osteoblasts and osteoclasts perform the continuous process of destroying old bone and creating new bone. Osteoclasts are the cells responsible for breaking down bone in need of remodeling, and osteoblasts are responsible for building it back up. This regenerative process is very slow, so slow in fact that it takes about seven years to regenerate the equivalent of a new skeleton. Osteoclasts are capable of breaking down bone 100 times faster than osteoblasts can rebuild it; however, while the body is young and growing, the osteoblasts do more than the osteoclasts, which leads to growth. But this cellular activity reaches a peak at around 35 to 40 years old, at which point the activity of the osteoclasts becomes greater than that of the osteoblasts. This flip in activity results in a gradual decrease in bone mass that continues until we die. This decrease is usually faster in women than in men and causes osteoporosis (porous bones) that result in spontaneous fractures, especially of the spine and hips.

Calcium hydroxyapatite

This is a naturally occurring mineral that makes up most of the mineral part of bone. It has the formula $Ca_5(PO_4)_3(OH)$. Hydroxyapatite is found our teeth and bones. In fact, it makes up about 90 percent of the surface layer of teeth called enamel and it is about 50 percent of our bones by weight. The OH group can be replaced by fluoride in the process of fluoridating water, making the enamel very hard and very resistant to tooth decay. Many modern implants, such as hip replacements and dental implants, are coated with hydroxyapatite to promote bone growth.

Bone consists of two quite different materials along with water. The first is called collagen, which is the major organic part of bone. The second material is a collection of bone minerals, the inorganic component of bone. Either of these components may be removed from bone and it will still have the shape of the original bone. The collagen remainder is quite flexible, somewhat like a chunk of rubber, and can even be bent into a loop. When the collagen is removed from the bone, the bone mineral remainder is very fragile and can be crushed with the fingers.

There are two types of bone: compact and spongy. Compact bone, while denser than spongy bone, is still hollow at the microscopic level. Blood vessels are seen in these hollow areas, which form major canals. These canals make the bone hollow. The compact bone is also rich with nerves, which cause pain when a bone is broken. Spongy bone has a greater surface area but is softer, weaker, and less dense and stiff than compact bone. It is typically found at the ends of long bones, near joints, and within vertebrae. Spongy bone contains red and yellow bone marrow. Red bone marrow is responsible for making red blood cells and, in the case of most adults, is located in the head of the femur and humerus. Yellow bone marrow is stored fat. When a bone is broken, this fat can be released into the blood and is capable of causing fatty clots that can be deadly.

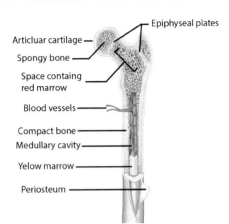

Finally there is the periosteum, a glistening double-layered tissue that creates a cover around compact bone. The periosteum is very thin and cannot be seen by the naked eye and is exceedingly important since it houses bone-forming osteoblast cells. The double layer also serves as a place where tendons and ligaments can insert and anchor into the bone.

Teeth

Teeth are a specialized type of bone. Given that teeth are white and tough it would be easy to assume that they are the same as bone, but this is not the case. The chemical composition of teeth can be better understood by breaking them down into their four major tissues: enamel, dentin, cementum and pulp.

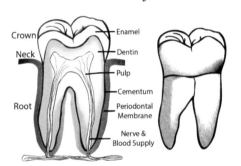

Enamel is the whitish covering of teeth and is the hardest substance in the entire body. About 96 percent of enamel consists of hydroxyapatite, compared to 50 percent of other bone throughout the body. Because of its high concentration of minerals, enamel is strong enough to withstand the stress of biting, chewing, and grinding. However, that same trait makes enamel more susceptible to chipping.

Dentin, a yellow-hued substance, makes up most of the tooth. It is responsible for giving the tooth its color. Because dentin is softer, it is more prone to decay.

Cementum, a yellowish substance covering the root of a tooth, is even softer than enamel and dentin. The role of the cementum is to help anchor the tooth to the jawbone and ensure its stability.

Dental pulp is the center part of the tooth that houses living connective tissue such as nerves and blood vessels.

The Strength of Bones

Healthy compact bone is able to withstand a compressive force of around 25,000 lb/in.[2] before it fractures. This means that the mid-shaft of the femur could support a force of around 12,000 lbs. or six tons.

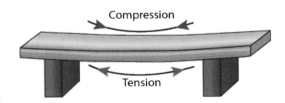

Femurs are very well designed and react to forces in a similar way to that of a beam in a building. In a beam, stresses cause it to pull apart on one side (tension) and push together on the opposite side (compression). The center of the beam experiences relatively little stress. This is why it is common to use I-beams in construction, as they have thick tops and bottoms joined with a thin midsection. In the case that the force comes from multiple directions, a hollow cylinder is used in order to achieve the maximum strength with a minimum amount of material, which is almost as strong as a solid cylinder of the same diameter. Since forces exerted on the femur may come from any direction, a hollow cylinder bone structure is appropriate. The compact bone of the shaft of the femur is thickest at the center. This is due to the fact that a hollow cylinder will buckle near the middle rather than at either end, much like if you push on one end of a soda straw.

The ability of bones to support the body's weight without breaking is crucial to human mobility and well-being. But bones support more than just the body's weight; they support other forces as well. For example, in bending over to pick up a heavy object we develop large forces on the lower spine. Large forces are also produced in activities such as running and jumping. When running, the forces produced on the hipbone when the heel strikes the ground can be up to four times the body's weight. Even walking creates forces on the hip around twice the body's weight. Due to the presence of these extra forces, bones must be exceedingly strong.

Breaking Bones

If bones are so strong and durable, then how do we produce forces that are strong enough to break them? The answer to this question is found in momentum. The mass, direction, and the velocity of an object determine its momentum; for

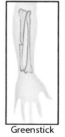
Intervertebral Disc

example, the bigger and faster an object is moving, the greater its momentum. A baseball flying through the air has a lot of momentum. When it hits a baseball bat, the force needed to change the baseball's direction (that is, its momentum) is huge and is done almost instantaneously. What this means is that the shorter the time of impact, the greater the force. In other words, what matters most is not how

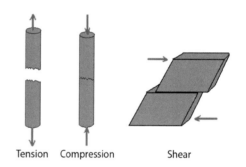
Tension   Compression   Shear

fast you are going when you stop, but how quickly you stop. So to reduce the force and thereby reduce the likelihood of a bone fracture, it is necessary to stop movement gradually. In a car this is done with shock absorbers. In a car accident it is accomplished by air bags and seat belts. In the human body, stopping gradually is accomplished in a number of ways. When a person jumps, he or she instinctively creates a system of shock absorbers through the bending of toes, ankles, knees, and hips. This bending motion is essential as it increases the time it takes to stop, thus decreasing the overall force on the body. Imagine if you jumped off a stool and landed on your heels without bending your knees. You would stop so abruptly that the force generated would be around 32,000 lbs., which is far greater than the force needed to fracture a femur. In addition to those already mentioned, there are other built-in shock absorbers. The discs in between the vertebrae are soft and cushiony and designed to absorb the forces of a rapid stop. The brain is supported on a platform called the tentorium, which is somewhat elastic and is surrounded by fluid, helping to protect the delicate structures of the brain from impact.

Fracture Types

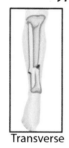
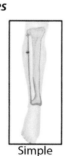
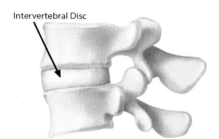

Greenstick (incomplete)   Transverse   Simple

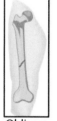
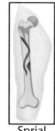
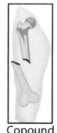

Oblique   Comminuted   Sprial   Copound

There are three ways that bones can break: tension, compression and shear. Bones do not normally break due to compression or tension; they are much more commonly broken due to shearing. A common cause of shear is catching the foot and then twisting the leg while falling. A shear fracture often results in a spiral break in which the bone is apt to puncture the skin. This type of fracture is called a compound fracture and is more likely to become infected than a simple fracture in which the bone is not exposed.

Questions – Chapter 10

1. What are the purposes that bones serve within the body? Explain each purpose.
2. What are the specialized cells involved in the construction and deconstruction of bone? Specify which cell performs which function.
3. What are the two types of bone?
4. Explain why bones are so strong.
5. Why do bones break? What is the most common type of fracture?

CHAPTER 11:

Voice Production

The human voice is an amazing tool that is used to create a variety of sounds such as whispering, speaking, shouting, laughing, crying, and singing. Generally, the way our voice sounds and how it is generated can be divided into three different parts. First, the process starts in the lungs, which is the source of the air needed to produce sound. The air then travels to the vocal folds in the larynx, which vibrate as the air passes producing sound. Finally, the air and sound travel to the articulators, which consist of the tongue, lips, and cheeks, and are used to modify even more the sound that is produced.

Step One: The Lungs

The first step of vocal production is found in the lungs. The lungs can be thought of as a pump that supplies needed air to the rest of the voice-producing mechanisms. The diaphragm muscle drives breathing. As air is exhaled and pushed outward it reaches the throat and trachea where the vocal folds and larynx are housed.

Step Two: The Vocal Folds

The vocal folds, also known as vocal cords, are located in the larynx and trachea. The larynx can also be called the voice box, and the trachea is the "breathing tube" in your body. The vocal folds are flat triangular bands that are attached to the trachea and larynx in the back (towards your spinal cord) as well as underneath the chin. Vocal folds are open while a person is breathing and are closed while swallowing. Air causes vocal folds to vibrate between open and closed positions when talking. Everyone has differently sized vocal folds with variations that cause our voices to be unique in their sound and pitch. This is what causes men to generally have lower voices while women have higher voices. It also causes singers to be grouped into different categories depending on the tone and pitch of their voices. Males have larger vocal folds that are about 17mm to 25mm in length, while females have vocal folds that are from 12.5mm to 17.5mm in length.

Sound is produced within the throat when the vocal folds vibrate as air passes through them, thereby changing the flow of air being expelled from the lungs. In order to produce higher-pitched sounds, they vibrate faster and have higher frequencies of up to 7000 Hz. To produce lower-pitched sounds, they vibrate slower with frequencies as low as 60 Hz. The process of converting the air pressure from the lungs into audible vibrations in medical terms is called "phonation" of voice production.

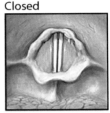

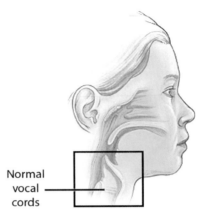

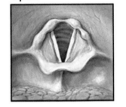

Closed

Open

Normal vocal cords

Step Three: The Articulators

Once the sound is made in the larynx and vocal folds, we must further manipulate the sound to articulate words and sounds by using our tongue, lips, and cheeks. These three parts, also known as the articulators, help produce recognizable words as the last step of the voice production system.

Voiced and Unvoiced Breath Sounds

There are 26 letters in the English alphabet, but there are 39 sounds (15 vowel sounds and 24 consonant sounds) produced by these letters. A **vowel** is a sound where air coming from the lungs is not blocked by the mouth or throat. All normal English words contain at least one vowel.

The vowels are **A, E, I, O, U and sometimes Y, which** can also behave as a consonant when it is at the beginning of a word. A consonant is a sound formed by stopping the air flowing through the mouth. The consonants are B, C, D, F, G, H, J, K, L, M, N, P, Q, R, S, T, V, W, X, Y, and Z. All the sounds produced in the English language are either voiced or voiceless. Voiced sounds occur when the vocal cords vibrate when the sound is produced. There is no vocal cord vibration when producing voiceless sounds such as whispering. Experiment with this by placing your fingertips on your throat as you create sounds. When saying the voiced sounds, you should be able to feel a vibration. When saying the voiceless sounds, you should not be able to feel a vibration. Sometimes it is very difficult to feel the difference between a voiced and an unvoiced sound. Another test may help. Put a piece of paper in front of your mouth when saying the sounds. The paper should move when saying the unvoiced sounds. All vowels in English are voiced. Some of the consonant sounds are voiced and some are voiceless. Some of the consonant sounds produced in English are very similar. Many times the difference between them is because one is voiced and the other is voiceless. Two examples are the letter "z," which is voiced, and the letter "s," which is unvoiced.

Voiced consonants: b, d, g, v, z, th, sz, j, l, m, n, ng, r, and w

Voiceless sounds: p, t, k, f, s, th, sh, ch, and h

Voice Disorders

Generally, the way we articulate our words and sounds come more naturally as we grow older. However, there are some disabilities and diseases that can affect the voice and how we produce sound. Vocal fold nodules or polyps may form on the vocal cords by misuse and injury and, if left untreated, can cause a hoarse, raspy voice and breathiness in individuals. Cancer may form in the larynx and throat, causing the vocal cords to be removed in the process of trying to get rid of the cancer. Also, there are speech and hearing disorders that affect how words and sounds are understood and repeated in our brains.

Some people have diseases and voice disorders from the time they are born. For example, dysarthria is a speech disorder resulting from neurological injury or resulting from underdevelopment. It causes a lack of coordination of tongue, lips, and throat. Some disorders are caused by physical abnormalities, such as a cleft palate, which changes the way sound comes out of an individual and how he or she pronounces and articulates sounds.

Questions – Chapter 11

1. What specific substance is needed in order to create sounds? (Hint: This does not include the organs included in the reading.)
2. Describe the process by which sound is produced by tracing the whole pathway.
3. What is the difference between voiced and unvoiced sounds?
4. What are some of the diseases and disabilities of the vocal pathway and their symptoms?

CHAPTER 12:
The Ear and Hearing

The ear converts very weak sound waves traveling through the air into electrical pulses on the auditory nerve that goes into the brain. However, what we commonly call the ear in reality does not refer to the visible part of the ear (the appendage we use to help hold up our eye glasses). This is called the pinna, and it is the least important part of the hearing system. It aids only slightly in funneling sound waves into the ear canal and can be completely removed with no noticeable loss of hearing. Many animals, including humans, have muscles to move the pinna. A horse has 17 muscles for each ear, while humans only have nine muscles. Most people do not have the nerve circuitry to activate these muscles. Those who do have control over the movement of these muscles can wiggle their ears. The part of the ear key to hearing is found inside the skull and is usually divided into three areas: the outer, the middle, and the inner ear.

The Outer Ear

The outer ear is a canal that begins at the opening of the skull and ends at the eardrum. It is also called the external auditory canal. This canal serves to increase the ear's sensitivity in the region of 3,000 to 4,000 Hz and also stores earwax. The canal is about 2.5 cm long (one inch) and is about the diameter of a pencil. You can think of the canal as an organ pipe closed at one end.

The eardrum, or tympanic membrane, is about 0.1 mm thick, which is paper-thin and has an area of about 65mm². It takes the vibrations in the air to the small bones in the middle ear.

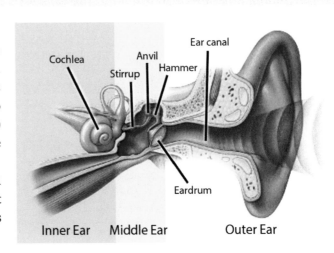

The Middle Ear

The dominant features of the middle ear are three small bones. These bones become mature size before birth. Thus the fetus can hear while it is still in the womb and will learn the sound of its mother's voice before being born.

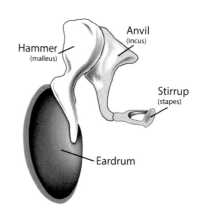

The bones are named after the objects they resemble: the malleus (hammer), the incus (anvil), and the stapes (stirrup). They are arranged so that they efficiently transmit vibrations from the eardrum to the inner ear. However, these bones do not transmit vibrations that they might pick up in the skull, such as those from your own voice. You hear your own voice primarily by transmission of sound through the air. Try plugging both your ears and listen to the reduction in sound volume of your own voice.

These bones change the vibrations of airwaves to vibrations of liquid waves in the fluid-filled chambers of the inner ear. They also considerably amplify sound. This sound amplification is accomplished in two ways. First, the place of connection between the eardrum and malleus is significantly larger than the area of the opening to the inner ear, called the oval window, where the stapes is connected. The difference in size amplifies the sound. The second way is through the action of lever arms. The attachment site for the malleus is off center, creating a lever. Then the other two bones are attached in such a way as to create additional levers. The combination of these two methods amplifies the sounds about 20 times. In fact, without the three bones of the middle ear, sound would simply bounce off the eardrum, with a person hearing hardly any sound at all.

Humans are much better at listening to soft sounds than we are at listening to loud sounds. In fact, loud sounds can damage the sense of hearing. The body has a muscle, called the stapedius muscle, which provides protection against loud sounds.

The Eustachian Tubes

The Eustachian tubes connect the middle ear to the back of your mouth. They serve as a drainage path for fluids generated in the middle ear. While they are closed most of the time, they can open momentarily, allowing the pressure in the middle ear to equalize with the atmosphere. The movement of the muscles in the face during swallowing, yawning, or chewing will usually cause a momentary opening of the Eustachian tube. Sometimes you hear a popping sound in one or both ears as the pressure equalizes and the eardrums return to their normal position. In babies the Eustachian tube is more horizontal, whereas in adults it becomes much more vertical. This makes it more difficult for babies to drain infection from the middle ear, so they are more prone to ear infections.

The Inner Ear

The inner ear is hidden deep within the skull, making it the best-protected sensory organ in the body. The inner ear contains the sensory organ for hearing, called the cochlea, and for balance, the vestibular system.

The snail-shaped cochlea is the organ that is dedicated to hearing by converting sound pressure waves from the outer ear into electrochemical impulses, which are passed on to the brain via the auditory nerve. It is filled with two fluids called the endolymph and perilymph. The Organ of Corti is the sensory receptor inside the cochlea, which holds hair cells that act as the nerve receptors for hearing. The mechanical energy from movement of the middle ear bones pushes in the oval window in the cochlea. This force moves the cochlea's fluids that, in turn, stimulate these tiny hair cells. The individual hair cells respond to specific sound frequencies (pitches) so that, depending on the pitch of the sound, only certain hair cells are stimulated. Signals from these hair cells are changed into nerve impulses. The nerve impulses are sent to the brain by the cochlear portion of the auditory nerve.

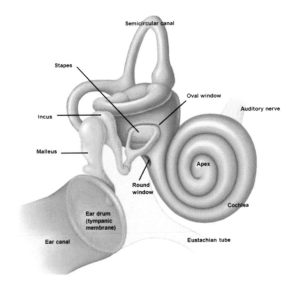

The vestibular system of the inner ear controls balance and is made up of the semicircular canals. These structures help control steadiness and balance with interaction between the eyes and feeling within the hands and feet. They send information to the brain about the relationship between the body and stationary surfaces in the environment. Sensors on the soles of the feet provide important information about the texture of the ground. This information is used to calculate weight and posture adjustments that will allow upright balance and movement. When people contract ear infections, they can become dizzy as the infection affects the vestibular system.

Diseases of the Ear and Hearing

Hearing Loss: The function of the external and middle ear is to collect and amplify sound. This system can fail in several ways and cause someone to become deaf or partially deaf. Hearing loss can be categorized into either the conductive or sensorineural type. Some patients experience mixed hearing loss, a combination of both types.

Conductive hearing loss occurs when the mechanical energy in the sound waves cannot be effectively transduced into the cochlea of the inner ear. The components responsible for the conduction of sound to the inner ear are the outer ear, outer ear canal, and tympanic membrane. Anything that obstructs the transmission of sound by these components or dampens the acoustic energy can result in conductive hearing loss. This type of hearing loss can often be corrected surgically, depending on the nature of the obstruction or malformation.

Sensorineural hearing loss occurs with damage to the cochlear apparatus, the sensitive hair cells in the inner ear that relay electrical signals to the brain, or in the auditory neurons within the central nervous system. Loud noise, viral infections, and specific drug side effects are often implicated in cases of damaged hair cells in the Organ of Corti. Age-associated hearing loss is of this type and can be treated with hearing aids, which simply amplify the sounds closest to the listener. This increases the sound input but does not improve clarity. In some cases, correction of sensorineural hearing loss can be achieved by a cochlear implant.

Questions – Chapter 12

1. What are the three major areas of the ear?
2. What are the two structures of the outer ear and what function does each of them serve?
3. Explain the two ways by which the three bones of the middle ear amplify sound before it travels to the inner ear.
4. What type of sounds are humans better at hearing?
5. Where do the Eustachian tubes run to and what is their main function?
6. How does sound change from a sound wave into a nerve impulse?
7. What are the two major parts of the inner ear and what are they responsible for?
8. How are humans able to balance on two feet?
9. Name the two types of hearing loss and the cause and effect of each.

Appendix A: Born to Run

The structure of our body has a lot to do with energy metabolism. They way we are built is a result of many years of evolution that created a structure to minimize energy needs while maximizing output. We as *Homo sapiens* evolved from *Homo erectus*, which was parallel to another species, Neanderthal. This species was superior in almost every aspect to the Homo erectus, but Neanderthal became extinct. So why did they go extinct, and why did we survive if we were the inferior species? The short answer is because Homo erectus stood upright whereas Neanderthal did not. You have seen pictures of them, hunched over, using all four extremities to walk and balance. The mere fact that we stand upright is not only the result of the need to hunt, breathe better, and transfer heat more easily from our bodies, but also because we could run better standing than we could by trying to do so on all fours. We as humans are born to run. It is in our DNA; it is in our nature. As Dr. Dennis Bramble, from the Department of Biology at the University of Utah, explains, "It is simple, just move your legs. Because if you don't believe that we are born to run, you're not only denying history. You're denying who you are."

So what makes us such great runners? Let's take a look at locomotion to better understand why being able to run is best when it comes to surviving.

To do this we have to go back thousands of years. It is here that we begin to understand how we were molded into the greatest distance runners the world has ever known. What allows us to be great marathoners are springy legs, twiggy torsos, sweat glands, hairless skin, and vertical bodies.

Regarding locomotion, mammals can be classified into two separate groups: runners and walkers. Runners are defined as mammals that run as part of their lifestyle, while walkers only run in an emergency. Examples of runners include tigers, horses, and dogs. Examples of walkers are pigs, cows, and chimps. In order to better understand the difference between walkers and runners, let's compare chimpanzees to humans. Chimps do not have an Achilles tendon and also have flat feet with long toes. We as humans possess an Achilles tendon and arched feet with short toes, both of which aid tremendously in running. Another key anatomical component that contributes to running is the gluteus maximus. Ours is large and muscular compared to that of a chimpanzee. What we as humans also posses is a nuchal ligament. This ligament is in the back of the neck and attaches to the base of the skull and assists in stabilizing the head when running. Walkers do not have a nuchal ligament, which makes it hard for them to run. If you ever see a pig try to run, it quickly becomes evident that it is awkward for it to run due to its head swaying uncontrollably.

Simply put, we have the perfect anatomy for endurance running.

We are not the fastest, but the engineering in our legs allows us to cover large distances. Important structures of our legs are as follows:

- High-volume capillaries for increased blood flow and oxygen exchange
- Rubbery tendons for high return of elastic energy

When you stand up, you lose thrust. So why do we stand upright? The main difference that we find when studying bipeds as opposed to quadrupeds is respiration rates. As quadrupeds run, each stride allows for only one breath. However, bipeds are able to breathe multiple times per stride. This plays a big part in running as it allows for increased oxygen exchange within the body. This is important as oxygen is needed in order to convert calories into energy.

We stand upright because we can run and we can run because we stand upright.

Another reason why respiration is so important is due to the fact that quadrupeds primarily cool down by breathing. Since quadrupeds heat up so quickly, they have to take frequent rests to cool down their body temperatures. If they do not rest, they overheat and are unable to continue moving, which can be fatal. However, for bipeds, that is the advantage of being able to sweat. We are able to cool off and run simultaneously. As long as we keep sweating, we can keep going. Standing upright allows for sweat to drip on our shoulders and evaporate, helping to take away excess heat.

Homo sapiens benefited from all of these anatomical structures over their Neanderthal counterparts. In fact, as the Ice Age came to an end it proved to be the reason the Homo sapiens survived and the Neanderthal perished. As forests began to dwindle, wildlife began to prosper on the open savannahs. This did not help the Neanderthals that relied so much on their long spears and ambush attacks—the animals were now able to anticipate such attacks. On the other hand, due to their ability to run, Homo sapiens took advantage of the climate shift and were able to hunt animals in a way that had never been seen before. They literally began to run animals to death. While it was not a fast process, Homo sapiens were able to focus on the anatomy of the quadrupeds to make them run until they overheated and died. It was due to this new hunting technique that we can see a change in the diets of the Homo sapiens from berries and fibrous plants to much more protein. They were finally able to hunt by outlasting animals.

So why do we not run as a people anymore? It simply comes down to the fact that our brains are the bargain shoppers of our bodies. The brain is always trying to find ways to save energy. Unlike any other organism, we have a conflict between our mind and our body. We have a body that is built purely for performance, but we have a brain that is all about the conservation of energy. For millions of years, we did not have reliable access to a steady supply of food. We relied on our legs for survival. As soon as we were able to have a steady and reliable source of food, our brains told us to rest and conserve our energy. While this may seem like an efficient decision, it also led to the decline of our natural-born calling.

Today our lifestyle has become a sedentary one, taking our high-performance bodies and placing them in an environment of leisure. Those people who have formed a habit of running know how good it feels to run. Once you lose the habit, your ancient survival instincts push you to relax. We have taken away the job that our bodies are meant to do. When astronauts first went into space it was thought that they would be healthier in the weightless environment of space. However, the opposite happened: they came back with aches and pains, depressed and ill, all due to the fact that they could not exercise and run. Anciently, we did not have many modern diseases such as diabetes or obesity. Now we are plagued with them. The way to prevent and even cure them is to do what our bodies were designed to do—run.

Appendix B: Magnetic Resonance Imaging

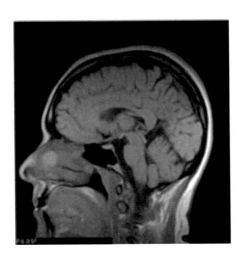

While X-rays do an excellent job of imaging bones, they aren't as good for imaging tissue. A better technique for studying tissue is *magnetic resonance imaging* or MRI. This technique locates hydrogen atoms by interacting with their magnetic nuclei. Since hydrogen atoms are common in both water and organic molecules, finding hydrogen atoms is a good way to study biological tissue.

It all starts when patients slide into an MRI machine, where they take with them the billions of atoms that make up the human body. For the purposes of an MRI scan, we're only concerned with the hydrogen atom, which is abundant since the body is mostly made up of water and fat. Each atom randomly spins, or precesses, on its axis, like a child's top. All of the atoms are going in various directions, but when placed in a magnetic field, the atoms line up in the direction of the field.

Since the magnetic field runs straight down the center of the machine, the hydrogen protons line up so that they're pointing to either the patient's feet or the head. About half go each way, so that the vast majority of the protons cancel each other out – that is, for each atom lined up toward the feet, one is lined up toward the head. Only a couple of protons out of every million aren't canceled out. This doesn't sound like much, but the sheer number of hydrogen atoms in the body is enough to create extremely detailed images. It's these unmatched atoms that we're concerned with now.

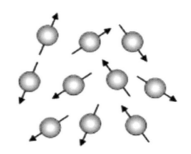

Next, the MRI machine applies a radio frequency (RF) pulse that is specific only to hydrogen. The system directs the pulse toward the area of the body we want to examine. When the pulse is applied, the unmatched protons absorb the energy and spin again in a different direction. This is the "resonance" part of the MRI. The RF pulse forces them to spin at a particular frequency and in a particular direction. The specific frequency that is used is calculated based on the particular tissue being imaged and the strength of the main magnetic field.

At approximately the same time, three gradient magnets jump into the act. They are arranged in such a manner inside the main magnet that when they're turned on and off rapidly in a specific manner, they alter the main magnetic field on a local level. What this means is that we can pick exactly which area of the body we want to image. This area is referred to as the slice. You can think of a loaf of bread with slices as thin as a few millimeters – the slices in MRI are that precise.

Slices can be taken of any part of the body in any direction, giving a huge advantage to MRI over any other type of imaging.

When the RF pulse is turned off, the hydrogen protons slowly return to their natural alignment within the magnetic field and release the energy absorbed from the RF pulses. When they do this, they give off a signal that the coils pick up and send to the computer system. The system goes through the patient's body point by point, building up a map of tissue types. It then integrates all of this information to create 2-D images or 3-D models with a mathematical formula known as the Fourier transform. The computer receives the signal from the spinning protons as mathematical data, and the data is converted into a picture. That's the "imaging" part of MRI.

Sometimes the MRI system uses injectable contrast, or dyes, to alter the local magnetic field in the tissue being examined. Normal and abnormal tissue respond differently to this slight alteration, giving us differing signals. An MRI system can display about 250 shades of gray to depict the varying tissue. The images allow doctors to visualize different types of tissue abnormalities better than they could without the contrast.

An MRI scanner is very noisy. It sounds a lot like a continual rapid hammering. That's due to the rising electrical current in the wires of the magnets being opposed by the main magnetic field. The stronger the magnet is, the louder the noise is.

Appendix C: Nutrition

Our bodies require a lot of energy, and an average human can consume thousands of calories each day to create that energy. However, it is important to fill our diets with the right kind of calories and not 'empty calories.' Examples of foods with empty calories are foods that have lots of sugars or solid fats, such as fried chicken, sugar-sweetened cereal, pizza, and whole milk. Many of these foods can be replaced with foods with 'better' calories that can supply energy and not add unneeded sugar and fat to our diets. Depending on what types of activities we are involved in during the day, we can consume more or less calories and still be considered healthy. For adult men and women, depending on age, weight, and gender, we should consume anywhere from 1600-2400 calories per day.

In order to have a healthy and balanced diet, we should eat foods from five different groups daily. These groups include fruits, vegetables, grains, proteins and dairy. Based on your weight, age, and gender, the amounts you should eat of each of these food groups can vary. For adult men and women, the website www.choosemyplate.gov suggests 1.5-2 cups of fruit, 2-3 cups of vegetables, 6-8 ounce equivalents of grains (3-4 ounces of these should be whole grains), 5-6 ounce equivalents of proteins, and 3 cups of dairy per day. An ounce equivalent of grain could be considered a half cup of cooked oatmeal, 2 small pancakes, or 5 whole wheat crackers. An ounce equivalent of protein could be considered 1 egg, ¼ cup of cooked beans, or 1 ounce of cooked lean beef. While oils are not considered to be a food group, they provide essential nutrients so they can be included in our diets; however, oils that are liquid at room temperature like olive oil, canola oil, and soybean oil are much better than oils that turn solid at room temperature like butter, shortening, and beef fats. The daily allowance of oils for adult men and women should be between 5-7 teaspoons. It should be remembered that these values are for individuals who get less than 30 minutes per day of physical activity and that those individuals who are more physically active may be able to consume more while staying within their caloric needs.

One diet that has had success and popularity in determining what types of foods that we should eat is the Mediterranean Diet. As the name suggests, it originated in the Mediterranean area and is based on food patterns of Greece and southern Italy. In addition to regular exercise and activity, it emphasizes abundant plant foods, fresh fruit as a typical dessert, olive oil as the principal source of fat, dairy products of cheese and yogurt, fish and poultry in low and moderate amounts, zero to four eggs (consumed weekly), and low amounts of red meat. Also, it calls for high consumption of legumes, unrefined cereals, fruits, and vegetables.

The reason for the use of olive oil as the principal fat is because it is made of monounsaturated fats that are easier for our bodies to break down and reduce the risk of heart disease. Many processed foods contain saturated and trans fats that cannot be broken down as well as unsaturated fats and are stored in higher amounts as fats in our body.

Adults should do 1 hour and 15 minutes of vigorous aerobic exercise per week to 2 hours and 30 minutes of moderate aerobic exercise per week. Adults should also do strengthening activities like push-ups, sit-ups and lifting weights at least 2 days a week. An average 154-pound male can burn 280 calories by walking for 1 hour and up to 590 calories while running for 1 hour.

Diets

Dieting has been used by many people over many years as a way of losing weight, maintaining fitness, and staying healthy. However, dieting is also used by athletes to gain weight and muscle in order to meet weight requirements. Whatever the case may be, diets can be effective if they are followed correctly and combined with other factors such as exercise and medicines.

Diets can be divided into some different categories, mainly low-fat diets, low-carbohydrate diets, and low-calorie diets. Some specific diets that fit into these categories will be discussed in this section. Because diets are mainly used for weight loss, a larger emphasis will be placed on diets that have been popular among the general public. In addition to limiting certain fats, carbohydrates, or calories, it is also important to remember that size and portion of snacks and meals are also important in dieting.

The Atkins diet is an example of a low-carbohydrate diet; it was created by Robert Atkins in the early 1970s. It focuses on limiting the consumption of carbohydrates in order to use the body's metabolism to use its stored fat as energy instead of the carbohydrates that normally would be consumed. This process is called ketosis, and as put by Dr. Atkins, "Burning fat takes more calories so you expend more calories." Another benefit claimed by this diet is that it helps to decrease the onset of hunger because fats and proteins generally take longer to digest than carbohydrates.

The South Beach diet, designed by Arthur Agatston and Marie Almon, serves as an alternative to other low-fat diets. The South Beach Diet can serve as a weight loss tool as well as a way to help prevent heart disease similar to other low-fat diets. The diet focuses on replacing 'bad' carbs and fats with 'good' carbs and fats. The bad carbohydrates mentioned are considered to be carbohydrate foods that the body digests quickly, creating a spike in blood sugar levels. They typically come from refined sugars and grains, whereas good carbohydrates are considered to be unprocessed foods like vegetables, beans, and whole grains that have a low glycemic index. The diet considers bad fat to be all trans fats and some saturated fats and tries to replace them with unsaturated fats and omega-3 fatty acids. These good types of fats come from lean meat, nuts, and oily fish.

Weight Watchers is an international company that offers products and services to assist in weight loss for registered members. The Weight Watchers program/diet is a type of low-calorie or calorie-limiting diet. Members are taught to lose weight by forming good habits of eating smarter and getting more exercise, and they are supported by others who have the same goals at member meetings. Foods are assigned point values based on the calories they contain. In order to lose weight to reach the goal weight, the individuals participating in the program only intake a certain amount of points each day.

Mediterranean Diet

This diet has turned into a very well known and acceptable diet for good lifelong health worldwide. The different aspects of this diet are as follows:

- A large amount of food should come from plant sources (where much of the protein comes from).
  - This includes vegetables, fruits, beans, seeds, nuts, and whole grains.
    - Grains, vegetables, and fruit should be eaten at most meals or whenever possible.
    - Vegetables may be cooked with olive oil, adding to the benefits of the diet, as long as the olive oil is used in moderation.
- Focus on consuming a variety of non-processed or minimally processed foods.
- Locally grown foods and seasonally fresh whole foods are also good choices.
- Use olive oil as the predominant fat in place of other fats like butter and margarine.
  - Extra virgin olive oil is healthiest in terms of fats and micronutrients.
- Low or moderate portions of cheese and yogurt should be consumed daily.
  - Types lower in fat are also good choices.
  - These are eaten regularly, but again, in small amounts.
  - These are important for bone and heart health.
- Fish and poultry should also be consumed in low to moderate amounts twice weekly.
  - Fish is high in omega-3 fats, making it preferable over poultry.
    - This will reduce the risk of heart disease and will also increase the immune system's functioning.
- Eat no more than seven eggs a week.
  - This includes those eggs used in baking.
  - Also, they should not be consumed mostly at the same time; try to space them out.
- Eat very small amounts of red meat.
  - Preferably you should eat only a couple or a few servings per month.
    - Types lower in fat would be good choices.
    - Poultry also makes a good substitute for this.
- Most desserts should consist mainly of fresh fruits.
- Consume wine in very moderate portions.
  - One to two glasses per day for men.
  - One glass per day for women.
  - This is only suggested if consumption is safe for the specific individual and for the people around that individual.
- Physical activity on a regular basis that promotes healthy weight and fitness levels.
- Overall, small amounts of saturated fat, sodium, sweets, and meat.
- Preparation is usually very simple for these foods.
- Moderation is key to this diet.

Although this is a very healthy diet, we know how hard it can be as a young college student to be able to adhere to these diets. Because of that, we have a few suggestions that will make it easier and less expensive for you to follow this diet.

1. It can be especially hard to consume the adequate amount of food from plant sources.
   a. To begin your day, fruit makes a wonderful addition to any breakfast.
   b. Vegetables should be consumed with both lunch and dinner.
   c. Vegetables also make great snacks in between meals.
   d. If you consume bread regularly in your meals, whole grain/wheat bread is a great choice.

2. Instead of cooking with butter and margarine, just use olive oil.
3. A great snack during the day is low-fat yogurt.
   a. A perfect addition to this is granola, which can make it easier for you to reach your goal of consuming enough plant foods.
   b. Cheese is also a good mid-day snack.
4. Instead of having red meat for dinner, which many of us tend to do, choose fresh fish or poultry.
   a. The more fresh the fish or poultry is, the better.
   b. And again, it is much healthier if you cook it with olive oil.
5. To get the adequate servings of eggs over the week, try to have one with your breakfast every couple of days.
   a. Also, try to reduce your amount of baked goods since eggs are used so extensively in these foods.
6. As mentioned earlier, try to substitute fish and poultry for red meat in your meals except for a few meals a month.
7. Dinner is a good meal with which to consume wine if you choose to do so.
   a. Again, only consume wine if it is safe for you and the people around you and if it follows your beliefs.
8. Instead of snacking on sweets during the day, snack on healthier foods like foods from plant sources and low-fat dairy foods.
9. And finally, be active.
   a. Walking is a great way to be active without actually going to the gym or on a run.
   b. Choose activities that you enjoy and that also provide you with adequate exercise.

Glossary

A

Acid reflux:	a condition in which gastric acid is regurgitated
Adenosine triphosphate (ATP):	an organic, phosphate-rich compound important in the transfer of energy in organisms
Adenosine diphosphate (ADP):	a compound of adenosine containing two phosphate groups, ADP is used to synthesize ATP with the energy released in cell respiration
Alpha particle:	a helium nucleus emitted by some radioactive substances, originally regarded as a ray
Alpha radiation:	ionizing radiation consisting of alpha particles, emitted by some substances undergoing radioactive decay
Alveoli:	any of the many tiny air sacs in the lungs where the exchange of oxygen and carbon dioxide takes place
Aneurysm:	an enlargement of part of the aorta that extends through the abdominal area and, at times, the upper portion of the aorta in the chest
Anode:	the positively charged electrode by which the electrons leave a device
Antimatter:	molecules formed by atoms consisting of antiprotons, anti-neutrons, and positrons
Aorta:	the main artery of the body, supplying oxygenated blood to the circulatory system
Aqueous:	of or containing water, typically as a solvent or a medium
Artery:	any of the muscular-walled tubes forming part of the circulation system by which blood (mainly that which has been oxygenated) is conveyed from the heart to all parts of the body
Asthma:	a chronic lung disease that inflames and narrows the airways, which causes recurring periods of wheezing, chest tightness, shortness of breath, and sometimes coughing
Astigmatism:	a defect in the eye or in a lens caused by a deviation from spherical curvature, which prevents light rays from meeting at a common point

B

Basal Metabolic Rate (BMR): the rate at which the body uses energy while at rest to keep vital functions going, such as breathing and keeping warm

Benign: mild and favorable

Beta: fast-moving electrons

Bile: a bitter greenish-brown alkaline fluid that aids digestion and is secreted by the liver and stored in the gallbladder

Bronchus: any of the major air passages of the lungs that diverge from the trachea

Bronchiole: any of the minute branches into which a bronchus divides

Bronchitis: a condition where the lining of the bronchial tubes becomes inflamed or infected, which reduces the amount of air that can flow into the lungs and causes mucus to form in the airways

C

Capillary: any of the fine branching blood vessels that form a network between the arterioles and venules; the smallest blood vessel

Carbohydrates: an organic compound that consists only of carbon hydrogen and oxygen

Carbon: the chemical element of atomic number 6, a nonmetal that has two main forms (diamond and graphite)

Cataract: cloudiness or opacity in the normally transparent crystalline lens of the eye. This cloudiness can cause a decrease in vision and may lead to eventual blindness

Cathode: the negatively charged electrode by which electrons enter an electrical device

Cementum: a specialized bony substance covering the root of a tooth

Chronic Obstructive Pulmonary Disease (COPD): destruction of the alveoli

Cilia: tiny hairs found on a cell or microscopic organism that beat rhythmically to aid the movement of a fluid past the cell or movement of the organism through liquid

Ciliary muscle: the smooth muscle in the ciliary body, the action of which affects the accommodation of the eye

Citric acid cycle: See **krebs cycle**

Cochlea: the spiral cavity of the inner ear containing the organ of Corti, which produces nerve impulses in response to sound vibrations

Collagen: the main structural protein found in animal connective tissue, yielding gelatin when boiled

Convection: the process of losing heat through the movement of air or water molecules across the skin

Cornea: the transparent layer forming the front of the eye

Cytomegalovirus: a kind of herpes virus that usually produces very mild symptoms in an infected person but may cause severe neurological damage in people

D

Dentin: hard, dense, bony tissue forming the bulk of a tooth beneath the enamel

Disaccharides: a complex sugar consisting of two linked monosaccharide units

E

Electron: a negatively charged particle surrounding the nucleus of an atom

Enamel: an opaque or semi-transparent glassy substance applied to metallic or other hand surfaces for ornamental purposes or as a protective coating

Energy: the capacity of a body or system to do work

Enzyme: any complex chemical produced by living cells that is a biochemical catalyst

F

Fats: energetically the most concentrated of all sustenance materials that are found in both plant and animal organisms, serving these living organisms as a source of energy

Fructose: fruit sugar occurs naturally in fruits, some root vegetables, cane sugar, and honey and is the sweetest of the sugars

G

Galactose: a six-carbon sugar that is a constituent of lactose

Gamma rays: penetrating electromagnetic radiation of shorter wavelength than X-rays

Glaucoma: a condition of increased pressure within the eyeball, causing gradual loss of sight

Glucose: a six-carbon monosaccharide produced in plants by photosynthesis and in animals by the metabolism of carbohydrates

Glycolysis: part of the metabolic process that includes the breakdown of glucose by enzymes, releasing energy and pyruvic acid; "the splitting of sugar"

H

Hemoglobin: the molecule found in the red blood cells that grabs onto oxygen and carries it in the blood

Hernia: a condition in which part of an organ is displaced and protrudes through the wall of the cavity containing it

Hydrocephalus: a condition in which fluid accumulates in the brain, typically in young children, enlarging the head and sometimes causing brain damage

Hydrogen: a colorless, odorless, highly flammable gas, the chemical element of atomic number 1

Hyperopia: also known as farsightedness

Hysterectomy: a surgical operation to remove all or part of the uterus

I

Ions: an atom or molecule with a net electric charge due to the loss or gain of one or more electrons

Ionizing radiation: radiation consisting of particles, X-rays, or gamma rays with sufficient energy to cause ionization in the medium through which it passes

Iris: a flat, colored, ring-shaped membrane behind the cornea of the eye, with an adjustable circular opening (pupil) in the center

K

Kinetic energy: energy that a body possesses by virtue of being in motion

Krebs cycle: the sequence of reactions by which most living cells generate energy during the process of aerobic respiration, which takes place in the mitochondria and converts ADP to ATP

L

Lactose: the naturally occurring sugar found in milk, formed by the combination of a molecule of galactose with a molecule of glucose

Lethal: harmful or destructive

M

Macula: an oval yellowish area surrounding the fovea near the center of the retina in the eye. It is the region of greatest visual activity

Macular degeneration: eye disease caused by degeneration of the cells of the macula lutea and results in blurred vision; can cause blindness

Malignant: (of a disease) very virulent or infectious

Maltose: formed during the germination of certain grains by the combination of two molecules of glucose

Membrane: a pliable sheet-like structure acting as a boundary, lining, or partition in an organism

Metabolism: the chemical processes that occur within a living organism in order to maintain life

Molecule: a group of atoms bonded together, representing the smallest fundamental unit of a chemical compound that can take part in a chemical reaction

Molybdenum: the chemical element of atomic number 42, a brittle silver-gray metal of the transition series, used in some alloy steels

Monosaccharides: a simple sugar such as glucose or fructose that cannot be broken down into simpler sugars

Myopia: also known as nearsightedness

N

Non-ionizing radiation: refers to any type of electromagnetic radiation that does not carry enough energy per quantum to ionize atoms or molecules

Nucleic acid: a complex organic substance present in living cells, especially DNA or RNA, whose molecules consist of many nucleotides linked in a long chain

Nucleus: the positively charged central core of an atom, containing most of its mass

O

Optic Nerve: each of the second pair of cranial nerves, transmitting impulses to the brain from the retina at the back of the eye

Orbital: a wave function describing the state of a single electron in an atom (atomic orbital) or in a molecule (molecular orbital)

Osteoblast: a cell that secretes the matrix for bone formation

Osteoclast: a large multinucleate bone cell that absorbs bone tissue during growth and healing

Osteoporosis: a medical condition in which the bones become brittle and fragile from loss of tissue, typically as a result of hormonal changes, long-term steroid therapy, and certain endocrine disorders

Oxidative phosphorylation: a vital process of intracellular respiration occurring within the mitochondria of the cell, responsible for most ATP production

P

Parathyroid hormone:	hormone synthesized and released into the blood stream by the parathyroid glands; regulates phosphorus and calcium in the body
Perfusion:	the process in which the right side of the heart pumps the entire blood supply of the body into the lung to exchange CO_2 for O_2
Periosteum:	a dense layer of vascular connective tissue enveloping the bones except at the surfaces of the joints
Pharynx:	The membrane-lined cavity behind the nose and mouth, connecting them to the trachea
Photons:	a particle representing a quantum of light or other electromagnetic radiation
Photoreceptor cells:	a photoreceptor, or photoreceptor cell, is a specialized type of neuron (nerve cell) found in the eye's retina
Plasma:	a nearly clear fluid like water, which is composed of clotting factors and immunoglobulins that help to fight infection
Pneumonia:	an infection of the lungs that is caused by bacteria, viruses, fungi, or parasites, which is characterized primarily by inflammation of the alveoli in the lungs or by alveoli that are filled with fluid
Pneumothorax:	a condition meaning "air in the chest" that can often be deadly
Positron:	a subatomic particle with the same mass as an electron and numerically equal but with a positive charge
Posterior:	further back in position; of or nearer the rear or hind end
Proteins:	a complex natural substance that has a globular or fibrous structure composed of linked amino acids
Pulp tissue:	the soft (not calcified) tissue in the pulp chamber; composed of blood vessels and nerves
Pupil:	the dark circular opening in the center of the iris of the eye, varying in size to regulate the amount of light reaching the retina
Refraction:	(in eyesight) has the ability to bend light rays entering it in order to focus them onto the retina
Rems:	the quantity of ionizing radiation whose biological effect is equal to that produced by one roentgen of x-rays
Retina:	a layer at the back of the eyeball containing cells that are sensitive to light and that trigger nerve impulses that pass via the optic nerve
Retinopathy:	a disease of the retina that results in impairment or loss of vision

S

Sclera: the white outer layer of the eyeball, continuous with the cornea at the front

Shadowgraph: a silhouette made by casting a shadow, usually of the hands, on a lighted surface

Sievert: International System of Units (SI) derived unit of equivalent radiation dose, effective dose, and committed dose

Sucrose: a disaccharide found naturally in many plants. Used in the production of sugar.

Surface tension: a property caused by attraction of molecules. It is responsible for many of the behaviors of liquids and allows liquid to resist an external force

T

Tentorium: a fold of the dura mater forming a partition between the cerebrum and cerebellum

Thorax: the part of the human body between the neck and abdomen, enclosed by the ribs and containing the heart and lungs; the chest

Trachea: a thin-walled, cartilaginous tube connecting the larynx to the bronchi; the windpipe

Tracheal rings: rings that support the airway, keeping it from collapsing when we exhale or when there is an absence of air

Tracheobronchial tree: the airway

Tumor: a swelling of a part of the body, generally without inflammation, caused by an abnormal growth of tissue, whether benign or malignant

Tungsten: the chemical element of atomic number 74, a hard steel-gray metal of the transition series

U

Ultraviolet: having a wavelength shorter than that of the violet end of the visible spectrum but longer than that of x-rays

Urethra: the duct by which urine is conveyed out of the body from the bladder, and which in male vertebrates also conveys semen

V

Ventricle: a fluid-filled cavity in the heart or brain

Ventilation: the process in which the airways provide oxygen to the lungs

Vitreous: like glass in appearance or physical properties

Voltage: an electromotive force or potential difference expressed in volts

W

Wavelength: the distance between successive crests of wave, especially points in a sound wave or electromagnetic wave

Z

Zonules: a small zone, band, or belt

Made in the USA
San Bernardino, CA
10 January 2017